MARCIA B. STEINHA...

S0-BYQ-406

16648196

Controversy
about
AMERICAN
HOSPITALS

Controversy about

AMERICAN HOSPITALS

Funding, Ownership, and Performance

J. ROGERS HOLLINGSWORTH

ELLEN JANE HOLLINGSWORTH

American Enterprise Institute for Public Policy Research
Washington, D.C.

J. Rogers Hollingsworth is professor of sociology and history and chairman, Program in Comparative History, University of Wisconsin. Ellen Jane Hollingsworth is the author and coauthor of books and articles on health and other social issues.

Distributed by arrangement with

UPA, Inc.
4720 Boston Way   3 Henrietta Street
Lanham, Md. 20706   London WC2E 8LU England

Library of Congress Cataloging-in-Publication Data

Hollingsworth, J. Rogers (Joseph Rogers), 1932–
    Controversy about American hospitals.

    (AEI studies ; 463)
    Includes index.
    1. Hospitals—economic aspects—United States.
    2. Hospital care—United States—Cost effectiveness.
    3. Hospitals—United States—Administration.
    I. Hollingsworth, Ellen Jane.   II. Title.   III. Series.
    [DNLM: 1. Economics, Hospital—trends—United States.
    2. Hospital Administration—trends—United States.
    3. Hospitals—United States.   4. Ownership—trends—United
    States.   WX 150 H741c]
    RA981.A2H55   1987   362.1'1'0973   87–19523
    ISBN 0-8447-3637-6 (alk. paper)
    ISBN 0-8447-3638-4 (pbk. : alk. paper)

1 3 5 7 9 10 8 6 4 2

AEI Studies 463

© 1987 by the American Enterprise Institute for Public Policy Research, Washington, D.C. All rights reserved. No part of this publication may be used or reproduced in any manner whatsoever without permission in writing from the American Enterprise Institute except in the case of brief quotations embodied in news articles, critical articles, or reviews. The views expressed in the publications of the American Enterprise Institute are those of the authors and do not necessarily reflect the views of the staff, advisory panels, officers, or trustees of AEI.

"American Enterprise Institute" and 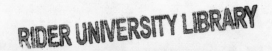 are registered service marks of the American Enterprise Institute for Public Policy Research.

Printed in the United States of America

RIDER UNIVERSITY LIBRARY

To Lauren, with love and devotion
and
To the memory of Walter Johnson

The American Enterprise Institute for Public Policy Research

Board of Trustees

Willard C. Butcher, *Chairman*
Chm. and CEO
Chase Manhattan Bank

Paul F. Oreffice, *Vice-Chm.*
Chm. and CEO
Dow Chemical Co.

W. Wallace Abbott
Senior Vice President
Procter & Gamble Co.

Robert Anderson
Chm. and CEO
Rockwell International Corp.

H. Brewster Atwater, Jr.
Chm. and CEO
General Mills, Inc.

Warren L. Batts
Chm. and CEO
Premark International

Winton M. Blount
Chm. and CEO
Blount, Inc.

Edwin L. Cox
Chairman,
Cox Oil & Gas, Inc.

John J. Creedon
Pres. and CEO
Metropolitan Life Insurance Co.

Christopher C. DeMuth
President
American Enterprise Institute

Charles T. Fisher III
Chm. and Pres.
National Bank of Detroit

D. Gale Johnson
Chairman
AEI Council of Academic
   Advisers

George M. Keller
Chm. and CEO
Chevron Corp.

Ben F. Love
Chm. and CEO
Texas Commerce Bancshares, Inc.

Richard B. Madden
Chm. and CEO
Potlatch Corp.

Founded in 1943, AEI is a nonpartisan, nonprofit, research and educational organization based in Washington, D.C. The Institute sponsors research, conducts seminars and conferences, and publishes books and periodicals.

AEI's research is carried out under three major programs: Economic Policy Studies; Foreign Policy and National Security Studies; and Social and Political Studies. The resident scholars and fellows listed in these pages are part of a network that also includes ninety adjunct scholars at leading universities throughout the United States and in several foreign countries.

The views expressed in AEI publications are those of the authors and do not necessarily reflect the views of the staff, advisory panels, officers, or trustees. AEI itself takes no positions on public policy issues.

Robert H. Malott
Chm. and CEO
FMC Corp.

Paul W. McCracken
Edmund Ezra Day University
   Professor Emeritus
University of Michigan

Randall Meyer
President
Exxon Co., U.S.A.

Paul A. Miller
Chm. and CEO
Pacific Lighting Corp.

Richard M. Morrow
Chm. and CEO
Amoco Corp.

James E. Olson
Chm. and CEO
AT&T

David Packard
Chairman
Hewlett-Packard Co.

Charles W. Parry
Director
Aluminum Co. of America

Edmund T. Pratt, Jr.
Chm. and CEO
Pfizer, Inc.

Mark Shepherd, Jr.
Chairman
Texas Instruments, Inc.

Roger B. Smith
Chm. and CEO
General Motors Corp.

Richard D. Wood
Chairman of the Board
Eli Lilly and Co.

Walter B. Wriston
Former Chairman
Citicorp

Officers

Christopher C. DeMuth
President

David B. Gerson
Executive Vice President

James F. Hicks
Vice President, Finance and
   Administration; Treasurer; and
   Secretary

Patrick Ford
Vice President, Public Affairs

Council of Academic Advisers

D. Gale Johnson, *Chairman*
Eliakim Hastings Moore
Distinguished Service Professor
of Economics
University of Chicago

Paul M. Bator
John P. Wilson Professor of Law
University of Chicago

Gary S. Becker
University Professor of Economics
and Sociology
University of Chicago

Donald C. Hellmann
Professor of Political Science and
International Studies
University of Washington

Gertrude Himmelfarb
Distinguished Professor of
History
City University of New York

Nelson W. Polsby
Professor of Political Science
University of California at
Berkeley

Herbert Stein
A. Willis Robertson
Professor of Economics
Emeritus
University of Virginia

Murray L. Weidenbaum
Mallinckrodt Distinguished
University Professor
Washington University

James Q. Wilson
James Collins Professor of
Management
University of California at
Los Angeles

Research Staff

Claude E. Barfield
Resident Fellow; Director,
Science and Technology

Walter Berns
Adjunct Scholar

Douglas J. Besharov
Resident Scholar; Director,
Social Responsibility Project

Nicholas N. Eberstadt
Visiting Scholar

Gerald R. Ford
Distinguished Fellow

Murray F. Foss
Visiting Scholar

Suzanne Garment
Resident Scholar

Allan Gerson
Resident Scholar

Robert A. Goldwin
Resident Scholar; Codirector,
Constitution Project

Gottfried Haberler
Resident Scholar

William S. Haraf
J. Edward Lundy Visiting Scholar;
Director, Financial Markets
Regulation Project

Karlyn H. Keene
Resident Fellow; Managing
Editor, *Public Opinion*

Jeane J. Kirkpatrick
Senior Fellow
Counselor to the President for
Foreign Policy Studies

Marvin H. Kosters
Resident Scholar; Director,
Economic Policy Studies

Irving Kristol
Senior Fellow

S. Robert Lichter
DeWitt Wallace Fellow

Chong-Pin Lin
Associate Director,
China Studies Program

John H. Makin
Resident Scholar; Director,
Fiscal Policy Studies

Brian F. Mannix
Resident Fellow; Managing
Editor, *Regulation*

Constantine C. Menges
Resident Scholar

Joshua Muravchik
Resident Scholar

Michael Novak
George F. Jewett Scholar;
Director, Social and Political
Studies

Norman J. Ornstein
Resident Scholar

Richard N. Perle
Resident Fellow

Thomas Robinson
Director, China
Studies Program

William A. Schambra
Resident Fellow; Codirector,
Constitution Project

William Schneider
Resident Fellow

Herbert Stein
Senior Fellow;
Editor, *AEI Economist*

Edward Styles
Director, Publications

Sir Alan Walters
Senior Fellow

Ben J. Wattenberg
Senior Fellow;
Coeditor, *Public Opinion*

Carolyn L. Weaver
Resident Scholar; Editor,
Regulation

John C. Weicher
F.K. Weyerhaeuser Scholar

Makoto Yokoyama
Visiting Fellow

Contents

LIST OF TABLES

Acknowledgments

We are indebted to many people who have assisted in various ways with the preparation of this manuscript. At the University of Wisconsin Burton H. Weisbrod sparked some of the initial thinking about nonprofit and public organizations, and throughout the project he has been responsive and helpful. On numerous occasions Jerald Hage and Robert Hanneman have provided useful advice about the study of complex organizations. Odin Anderson has been a constant source of information about American hospitals and kindly read the entire manuscript. Others who read the manuscript and made helpful comments were Pat Arnold, Marion Lewin, Jack Meyer, and Steven Sieverts. We are also very grateful to Andy Aoki and Dan Bailey for their very valuable research assistance on the project.

The Program on Non-Profit Organizations at Yale University provided initial funding for the project, and John Simon and Paul DiMaggio, also of Yale, offered invaluable advice at every stage. Indeed, without their assistance, the project might never have been completed. We are also very grateful to the American Enterprise Institute and the Klingenstein Fund of New York for providing financial support for the research and publication of our manuscript. At the University of Wisconsin the Graduate Research Committee made funding available for various aspects of the project, and the Institute for Research on Poverty supplied computer programming assistance. We are also grateful to the American Hospital Association and to the director of its data center, Dr. Ross Mullner, for providing data tapes of various hospital surveys. Others who helped to make the study possible by providing data or strategic advice were Montague Brown, William S. Custer, Bradford Gray, Frank Sloan, Daniel Wikler, and Rosemary Stevens.

To thank the dozens of hospital administrators who consented to be interviewed would require extensive listing. Suffice it to say that their perspectives have been invaluable. No amount of published literature can provide the rich insights that hospital, state hospital association, and state regulatory personnel have given to this book.

Many librarians in small towns in southeastern, midwestern, and mountain states generously shared materials with us.

We especially want to thank Sandy Heitzkey and Jane Mesler of the Department of History at the University of Wisconsin for arranging for the typing of several drafts of the manuscript, always in a very cheerful and efficient manner.

1
Introduction

Medical care in the United States cost about $400 billion in 1985. It is big business and the subject of great controversy. During the past decade the hospital, as part of the medical system, has become the focus of much of the controversy. Attention has centered on how to control hospital costs, the large-scale activities of for-profit corporations in providing medical care, the extent to which alternative payment systems for Medicare might alter hospitals' behavior, and how the nation can provide needed hospital services for the 35 million people who do not have hospital insurance of any kind. Increasing concern has emerged about the extent to which the intense businesslike orientation of hospitals of all kinds has undermined their role as community institutions providing a much-needed public service. Although many other serious issues exist, these have engendered the most discussion.

This study is concerned primarily with comparing the behavior of for-profit, public, and voluntary hospitals. The charges and countercharges often heard in the debate about these three kinds of hospitals include the following:

• Investor-owned hospitals use resources more efficiently, are cost efficient, have easier access to capital, and lower the costs of medical care.

• Investor-owned hospitals engage in cream skimming and dumping of poor patients while public and voluntary hospitals provide more care for the poor.

• Nonprofit hospitals (public and voluntary) provide higher quality, easier access to care, and lower-cost care than investor-owned hospitals.

• Physicians in voluntary hospitals enjoy more professional autonomy than physicians in either public or for-profit hospitals.

• The entire hospital industry has become commercialized, and the behavior of voluntary and public hospitals is increasingly like that of investor-owned hospitals.

The defenders of each kind of hospital have often been very shrill. Partly as a result, the behavior of hospitals in the three sectors is

1

poorly understood by consumers. Thus a major purpose of this book is to provide information on the different ways that hospitals in these three sectors behave and to explain why the United States, unlike most countries, has many hospitals of all three kinds. A major issue is to understand for the entire twentieth century the conditions under which the behavior of hospitals in these three sectors has diverged and the conditions under which it has converged. The study will address the issue of whether the type of ownership has made any difference in costs, efficiency, quality, accessibility, and responsiveness to community need.

Because no discipline has a monopoly on the problems addressed here, we borrow theoretical insights from varied sources. Some may object to an analysis that is not derived deductively from a single rich body of theory. Many studies demonstrate, however, that knowledge is often advanced and new insights are developed when scholars attempt to integrate diverse theories.[1] It is in this spirit that this study is deliberately eclectic. It borrows from a diverse literature in economics and sociology but is primarily a historical study focusing on the structure and behavior of hospitals throughout the twentieth century.

Economists have long attempted to model the behavior of public and for-profit organizations, but only in recent years have they begun to make substantial headway in understanding the nonprofit sector[2] and the economics of altruism.[3] Efforts have been made to relate the theoretical literature on nonprofit organizations to contemporary analysis of hospitals, but so far little effort has been made to integrate the insights of studies on the nonprofit sector with the economics of industrial organization and the sociology of complex organizations. This study makes some modest attempt to speak to these issues within a historical context.

The organizational literature may be placed in two broad categories. One category is concerned with understanding how the environment of organizations limits their structure and behavior. Here one thinks immediately of the work of industrial organizational economists such as Caves and Williamson, institutional economists such as Nelson, Davis, and North, and organizational sociologists such as Aldrich, Freeman, Hannan, Lawrence, and Pfeffer.[4] Their work emphasizes how the following environmental variables limit what kinds of organization may emerge and how they behave: rates of change in technology, technological complexity, heterogeneity or homogeneity of demand, the availability of resources, and private and public regulation.

Organizational forms are not shaped exclusively by external vari-

2

ables, however. Within organizations the perception and cognition of actors also shape structure and behavior. The work of Argyris, Lawrence, March, and Simon comes to mind.[5] These scholars have studied decision making to understand the critical choices that organizations make.

This study speaks to both these traditions in the organizational literature and attempts to show how specific environments gave rise to public, voluntary nonprofit, or for-profit hospitals. Unfortunately, most of the scholarly literature that has analyzed environmental effects on organizations has been cross-sectional and rather static. By undertaking a historical analysis of American hospitals, however, this study is able to suggest how changes in the environment influenced changes in the structure and behavior of hospitals in the three sectors. Finally, the study confronts the question of how the form of organization (that is, the type of ownership) influenced the decisions made within hospitals. That is, to what extent do decision makers in public hospitals pursue different goals and have different perceptions about the nature of hospitals from those held by decision makers in voluntary nonprofit and for-profit hospitals?

For the period between 1830 and 1940 Alfred Chandler, in several brilliant histories of American manufacturing and transportation firms, has provided a convincing explanation of why specific firms became nationwide corporations and the conditions under which they developed either a highly centralized organization along functional lines or the more decentralized multidivisional (M-form) structure. Very few studies have been made, however, of the development of organizations in the service sector, especially organizations in the voluntary nonprofit and public sectors. Hence an important concern of this study is to address the extent to which recent changes in the history of American hospitals correspond to the histories of the manufacturing sectors. Chapter 4 addresses some of the tensions that have arisen as the hospital industry has become more like others in the American economy.[6]

Hospitals are an ideal subject for understanding how a service industry operating in these three sectors behaves over time; few areas of the American economy, particularly during the twentieth century, provide such excellent data. By analyzing American hospitals over time within the framework of the bodies of literature discussed above, we hope to shed light on why the American hospital industry is changing so rapidly.

This study is a history of American hospitals during the twentieth century. Before presenting our specific findings, however, we

3

discuss some of the generalizations developed in the study. (For a discussion of the concepts and data underlying the study, consult the Appendix.)

Origin of Twentieth-Century Hospitals:
Trust, Heterogeneity of Demand, and Availability of Capital

Before 1900 most Americans, when seriously ill, preferred to be—indeed, expected to be—treated at home. Not only could hospitals do little to treat most patients, but few hospitals existed. As hospitals developed in the United States, public and voluntary hospitals enjoyed much greater legitimacy than those in the for-profit sector. Americans have historically preferred to provide goods and services in the for-profit sector, but Kenneth Arrow, Burton Weisbrod, and others have reminded us that medicine has developed somewhat differently.[7] Briefly, for some sectors of the economy markets are poorly equipped to coordinate services between providers and consumers. Many people have placed hospitals in such a category, despite the many for-profit hospitals in the American past.

It is often suggested that it is unethical for hospitals to earn money from the illness of others. But Arrow's argument is more cogent. When consumers have lacked sufficient information to control and judge the quality of a product, they have feared exploitation by for-profit organizations and have therefore sought the safeguard of the nonprofit organization. Although private medical and dental practices and the manufacture of pharmaceutical drugs have also been characterized by gross discrepancies in the knowledge possessed by suppliers and consumers, considerable public and private regulation has assured consumers that they can trust providers. For-profit hospitals have historically suffered from a lack of legitimacy, although the regulatory environment of the past two decades has helped them to overcome distrust among consumers. But this historical distrust was one of the most important reasons why the for-profit hospital did not become the dominant pattern in the United States or in any other country. Of course, the growth of for-profit hospitals has been constrained in the United States for other major reasons: they have avoided providing unprofitable collective goods, such as teaching, research, and emergency care; and they have had little incentive to serve charity patients or other unprofitable groups.

Although most Americans before 1900 preferred to be treated at home, there were always others, travelers and the poor, for example, who needed hospitals. Responding to these needs, society early made some effort to provide public or voluntary hospitals.

4

If everyone had had the same preference, with equal intensity, about what kind of hospitals should exist, most hospitals might have emerged in the public sector, but groups had differing preferences and with differing intensities about the functions hospitals should serve. Thus various minorities founded voluntary hospitals to address specific needs; that is, they were willing in numerous cities to support a hospital that would offer specific services for which there was not a demand from a majority of the citizens. Donors in the late nineteenth and early twentieth centuries generally provided support for others somewhat similar to themselves, though customarily favoring those below themselves in status and income. Historically, it was ethnic and religious diversity that gave rise to a sizable voluntary sector in America, whereas countries with very homogeneous populations (such as Sweden, Denmark, and Norway) have developed public hospitals.

Not all American minorities, of course, had the same capacity to provide hospitals. First, and most important, a minority had to have available capital. Some ethnic and religious groups could not build hospitals because they lacked financial resources. Even if capital was available, whether a minority could mobilize sufficient funding for a hospital, particularly a large hospital, depended on the cohesiveness of the group—the amount of its interaction, the degree of familiarity among its members, the homogeneity of opinion within it, and the importance of a hospital to it. With strong group cohesion individual group members derived a sense of identification, gratification, and pleasure from engaging in philanthropic activity.[8]

Because group cohesion was so important, it is significant that capital was generally raised locally for a specific community hospital. Large groups that transcended or encompassed many cities generally lacked the cohesion to support a community hospital. Until recent years voluntary hospitals were very much integrated into the communities of which they were a part and attempted to serve those communities in exchange for support. Some scholars stress that the term "community hospital" has often been more invention than reality.[9] To some extent Catholic hospitals in the United States were an exception, however. Although they were generally integrated into their communities, they also received substantial extracommunity support from dozens of religious orders that raised money from diverse sources.

While voluntary nonprofit hospitals emerged in cities where ethnic and religious minorities had intense and strong group consciousness, the public sector was more responsive to majoritarian interests, responded to community needs that were not met by the voluntary sector, and provided facilities that met a lower standard of

5

acceptability. The public sector has historically provided services about which there is a widely shared consensus in a community—or in response to what some have called the demands of the median voter. In many large cities of the nineteenth and early twentieth centuries, for example, the "undeserving poor" were not served by the voluntary sector, and the public hospital attempted to meet their needs. In other cities that had no distinctive minorities with sufficient capital to develop voluntary hospitals, the state could raise the revenue for a public sector hospital through taxation. That is, in many cities people wanted a hospital but were not prepared to bear the costs voluntarily. Thus, in many smaller cities, particularly where the population was relatively homogeneous religiously and ethnically, public hospitals emerged.

Many cities early in their development lacked sufficient capital for hospitals in either the public or the voluntary sector; still there was some demand for hospitals. In such communities—especially during the first third of this century—for-profit hospitals were often established by physicians or surgeons as appendages to their private practices. These hospitals served the specific needs of physicians and their patients, were small, required little capital, and provided a narrow array of services.

Early in the twentieth century hospitals in these three sectors had quite diverse sources of capital and rather different sources of income. Because hospitals were responsive to the preferences of those who provided resources, their behavior varied greatly from sector to sector. Voluntary hospitals were constrained by the preferences of the philanthropic groups that contributed to their development and maintenance, although in time some began to rely on public subsidies, especially for the treatment of the poor, and almost all had to rely to some extent on paying patients. Public hospitals were much more constrained by the imperatives of public authorities, although in time most of them also depended to some extent on paying patients. The private for-profit hospitals received almost all their income from private paying patients and provided somewhat more individualized care than hospitals in the two other sectors.

Persistence

Once established, public and voluntary hospitals tended to persist. Providing a valued but increasingly costly service, they could not continue to rely solely on traditional sources of revenue. Philanthropy continued to provide support for many voluntary hospitals, but patients' payments first augmented and then overwhelmed philanthropy. If a particular ethnic or religious group established a hospital, the hospital could generally depend on the group for financial support for many years. In public hospitals governmental authorities continued to provide support, but patients' fees increasingly became a substantial proportion of revenue. Sunk costs in both public and voluntary nonprofit hospitals also contributed substantially to their survival rates.

The situation was quite different for for-profit hospitals, however. They did not enjoy the same legitimacy as nonprofit or public hospitals, and their survival was much more dependent on a single individual. When physicians who established proprietary hospitals died or retired, the hospitals often closed or were transformed into public or nonprofit hospitals, the outcome depending on the developmental stage of the community, the availability of capital, the ethnic and religious heterogeneity of the community, and the demand for a hospital. Survival rates of for-profit hospitals were much lower than those of public or voluntary hospitals.

Changes in the Sources of Operating and Capital Revenues

As the demand and the costs of hospital care increased, the public and philanthropic sectors could not provide all the daily maintenance costs for patients. Because the United States did not develop a system of national health insurance, as a number of European societies did, patients had to finance a rising share of their hospital costs. As a result private health insurance began to grow rapidly during the 1930s. By the end of the 1950s, it had become pervasive, although many persons, particularly the poor and the elderly, remained without medical insurance.

During the interwar period hospitals had continued to grow in response to patients' demands. They were mostly financed by cities, but some communities simply lacked adequate funds with which to construct hospitals. Given the uneven funding and the distribution of medical insurance, U.S. society had by 1946 almost reached its capacity to construct hospitals, without some alternative means of supplying capital. That year Congress passed the Hill-Burton Act to stimulate the construction of hospitals in areas that needed them but lacked the capital to finance them. With federal money available, many cities for the first time had sufficient capital to construct hospitals. Since federal money had to be matched with local money and was generally a "one-shot" infusion, hospitals continued to be controlled locally. As a result of the Hill-Burton Act, hospitals, especially small hospitals, dramatically increased during the next quarter-century.

The Hill-Burton program reflected the prejudices of American society against for-profit hospitals, which were not eligible to receive Hill-Burton funds. The proportion of hospitals in the for-profit sector declined substantially after 1946, reaching an all-time low during the early 1970s. Early in the twentieth century cities without adequate public or philanthropic funding had often developed hospitals in the for-profit sector; after the enactment of the Hill-Burton program, many cities in this situation could acquire federal funding for the construction of public or nonprofit hospitals.

Availability of Resources and an Expanding Industry

Even though most cities could afford hospitals as a result of Hill-Burton funding, by 1960 a sizable segment of the U.S. population was unable to afford hospital care. Congress addressed this problem in 1965 by enacting the Medicare and Medicaid programs to increase access to hospital care for the elderly and the poor. Unlike the Hill-Burton program, the Medicare and Medicaid funds did not discriminate against for-profit hospitals; physicians and patients could choose among hospitals. With the infusion of these funds, the demand for hospital services suddenly increased, and the numbers of hospitals and beds in all three sectors expanded.

The reimbursement policies of the Medicaid and Medicare programs vastly enhanced the prospects for survival of for-profit hospitals. They became subject to many of the same public and private regulatory authorities as public and voluntary nonprofit hospitals, which enhanced their legitimacy despite longstanding suspicion and distrust.

During the mid-1960s increasing access to hospitals was a central concern of the U.S. government; budgetary concerns were then relatively unimportant. With ineffective controls on spending, expensive and complex technology rapidly diffused to hospitals in all three sectors. By the end of the 1970s many observers believed that the entire hospital industry had become overbuilt and inefficient. The average size of a hospital was 150 beds, about half the size many experts believed necessary for efficient operations.

As the U.S. hospital industry expanded and its costs increased, society slowly reversed its priorities. It became more concerned with cost containment and less concerned with access to hospitals. In an effort to contain costs, state and federal governments had enacted a variety of regulatory programs by 1980. In most industries a major purpose of regulation is to reduce uncertainty by stabilizing competition. In the hospital sector, however, the purpose of much regulatory legislation was to introduce the restraints on spending that existed naturally within firms in most sectors of the economy. Because of third-party reimbursement, the hospital industry differed from most sectors of the American economy; hospitals had little incentive to contain costs. Much of the hospital regulation of the 1970s was designed to control costs by eliminating the technical inefficiency due to excess capacity and unnecessary duplication.[10]

Resource Constraints and Structural Change

By the mid-1970s the environment of U.S. hospitals had become extraordinarily complex. First, there was a vast diversity of third-party payers. Second, there were numerous regulatory bodies—local, state, and federal, as well as private. Third, although in the early twentieth century hospitals had raised most of their capital locally through philanthropy and the public purse, the sources of capital became much more diverse after the Hill-Burton, Medicare, and Medicaid programs were enacted. Hospitals turned increasingly to the federal government for capital as well as to global capital markets. As hospitals became less dependent on their communities for capital, they also became less integrated into community affairs. Their internal structure also became much more differentiated.

Hospitals also began to respond to other environmental changes. Technological change, for example, shifted many kinds of surgery and other services that for decades had taken place in hospitals to alternative sites. With substitutes for hospitalization, overcapacity began to be a serious problem in many parts of the country. Large purchasers of medical care were meanwhile beginning to use their market power to lower hospital use and costs.[11]

Alfred Chandler has demonstrated through the histories of various manufacturing sectors that industries with overcapacity combined with the potential to develop economies of scale have undergone substantial consolidation. That combination led to consolidation in the U.S. hospital industry during the 1970s and 1980s. The pressure on hospital costs has also been a pronounced factor in inducing consolidation. Without that pressure the hospital industry's sensitivity to economies of scale would have been much less.

Consolidation in an industry takes the form of either a loose coupling among firms or tight integration. Both kinds of consolidation have occurred in the U.S. hospital industry. Loose coupling has occurred when hospitals determined to maintain their separate autonomy have joined together in multihospital systems to confront one or two major problems—to exploit economies of scale in shared purchasing or in shared billing, for example. Other hospitals have resorted to mergers to attain tighter and more effective controls, as well as economies of scale, over a host of activities: purchasing, cost accounting, billing, the costs of capital, insurance, legal services, and so on.

As the external environment of hospitals has become increasingly differentiated, large hospitals have had a somewhat greater capacity to develop internal specialized expertise to cope with their environments than free-standing, small hospitals. Even very large, independent, free-standing hospitals have had a somewhat limited capacity, however, to respond to the rapidly changing, increasingly unstable environment. During the 1970s and early 1980s those that have coped most effectively with their environmental uncertainties have been the investor-owned hospitals that have gone through extensive horizontal mergers and have become part of highly differentiated systems. By operating on a large enough scale, some hospital systems have developed a highly specialized managerial hierarchy capable of coordinating, monitoring, and planning for many separate hospital units. Whether in the nonprofit or the for-profit sector, complex managerial hierarchies acquired the specialized skill to handle effectively the complicated legal problems of the nation's fragmented regulatory climate and capital markets. By developing complex information systems, well-differentiated managerial hierarchies have been able to exploit economies of scale and to improve their cash flows.

The hospital industry, however, cannot develop the economies of scale of the steel, automobile, or food-processing industries (or other industries using a relatively standardized technology to produce standardized products); in the hospital industry technology changes too rapidly, and there is no standardized therapy for all problems.[12] Hospital organizations that have directed their activities to a relatively narrow array of markets have had a greater capacity to consolidate and to develop economies of scale than those that—for whatever reason—have attempted to serve a broader array. In short, the three hospital sectors have varied in their capacities to become consolidated in tightly integrated systems and therefore in their capacities to develop specialized managerial hierarchies.

Investor-owned hospitals have had the greatest flexibility to change their structure and to merge into larger, tightly controlled organizations. Primarily attempting to maximize profits, the managers of investor-owned hospitals have believed that they could best enhance their efficiency and productivity by developing chains of hospitals. Some of these organizations have taken on the multidivisional structure (M-form structure) that Chandler and Williamson have shown is the dominant form for American firms once they reach a certain size and complexity. Within the M-form organization, a national or international office plans long-term strategy for a system of hospitals and allocates capital to various parts of the organization, while those in managerial positions at the local hospital are concerned primarily with its day-to-day problems. Once a hospital organization has adopted the M-form structure, it has substantial capacity to increase its size, to add more hospitals, to operate in diverse geographical markets—even foreign ones—and to move into other product lines.[13]

Of the three kinds of hospitals, the public hospital has had the least capacity to lose its autonomy by merging into a larger organization. Whereas the dominant goal of the investor-owned hospital has been to earn profits, public hospitals have many more socially defined objectives. The investor-owned hospital has had much greater flexibility to close, to expand, or to restrict its services, but most public hospitals have been tied to a specific community and subject to many social constraints. As a result, many public hospitals, especially the larger ones, have attempted to serve more heterogeneous markets that are not profit oriented (burn centers, trauma centers, teaching units) than investor-owned hospitals. In contrast to the large, urban public hospital, small public hospitals—especially those in small towns and rural areas—have had fewer constituencies to serve and greater capacity to close, to change their type of ownership, or to merge into larger organizations.

The capacity of the voluntary nonprofit hospital to become consolidated into larger organizations has lain between that of the public and the investor-owned hospital. Voluntary hospitals have had more socially defined objectives than investor-owned hospitals, but their flexibility has been constrained by local groups to which they have attempted to be responsive. Many such hospitals have come on difficult times.

Voluntary hospitals in many large cities came into existence in response to the demands of ethnic or religious groups that have become less ethnically or religiously conscious. Often they have moved to the suburbs, leaving their hospitals behind without strong community support.

Meanwhile, because of Medicare and Medicaid reimbursement policies, philanthropic giving to voluntary hospitals has substantially declined; as a percentage of all hospital construction costs, it declined

11

by 54 percent between 1964 and 1975. Indeed, by the 1980s the proportion of capital and operating expenses derived from philanthropy had reached its lowest point in the twentieth century—even lower than during the depression of the 1930s.[14]

It has also become increasingly difficult for voluntary hospitals to finance capital improvements from internal funds or local governmental revenues. Like investor-owned hospitals, they have found it necessary to turn to the capital markets. But those markets are very sensitive to the following indicators in granting attractive financing to hospitals: the quality of management, the geographical location, the occupancy rate, the average length of stay of patients, the profitability, the debt-asset ratio, the share of the local market, and the local regulatory environment. Voluntary and public hospitals are very much constrained by sunk costs, however, and therefore have somewhat less capacity than investor-owned hospitals to change their structure so as to rank high on these indicators.

Because of the substantial changes in their environment, many voluntary hospitals have successfully resorted to a loose coupling arrangement to achieve specific economies of scale. The tightly managed, integrated chains that have become common in the for-profit sector have also occurred, but less frequently in the voluntary sector.

Whether consolidation takes the form of loose coupling or of tight integration, most hospital consolidation has been horizontal; the vertical integration that has occurred in a number of manufacturing sectors has been less common. A major incentive for vertical integration in other industries has been to lower transaction costs, to achieve economies of scale, and to reduce uncertainty in their environment.[15] The potential to do so is less in the hospital industry than in the steel, oil, aluminum, and other industries in which vertical integration has been extensive.

Of course, some efforts toward vertical integration have been made in both the voluntary nonprofit and the for-profit sectors. In an effort to maximize their supply of patients, for example, hospitals have acquired intermediate- and long-term-care facilities and have developed such other facilities as satellite hospitals, free-standing ambulatory centers, and hospital transportation facilities. A few hospitals have developed their own health maintenance organizations (HMOs), while others have formed close contractual relations with HMOs or other third-party payers. Most vertical integration has been local, however. A hospital in one city has little incentive to construct a doctor's office or to own a pharmacy in another city. Because the hospital industry has so many production centers (hospitals), it is unlikely that vertical integration will become as extensive as in the steel, oil, aluminum, or other industries, which have relatively few production centers. And while vertical integration is likely to continue developing in the American health industry, there are numerous indications that hospitals will also resort to alternative strategies for relating to other actors in the health area. For example, a great deal of informal networking, long-term contractual relations outside a single organization, is emerging. This kind of loose relationship among various actors permits far more flexibility among hospitals and other health organizations than the strategy of vertical integration.

Source of Funding, Performance, and Behavior of Hospitals

The behavior and performance of hospitals in the three sectors have exhibited distinct differences. These have been most pronounced when hospitals in the three sectors have received their funding from distinct sources and least pronounced when their sources of funding have converged. Different sources of funding cause different behavior because the sources are tied to groups with distinct preferences that shape that behavior.

In the early twentieth century hospitals in the three sectors received most of their funding from distinctly different sources. For-profit hospitals received most of their funding from paying patients or from the for-profit sector, public hospitals from the public sector. The voluntary nonprofit hospitals received substantial sums from the voluntary sector, although they also received funds from the public sector and from paying patients.

Histories of hospitals and literature in numerous journals suggest that early in the twentieth century hospitals that received funding from distinctly different sources tended to behave as shown in table 1.[16] Because public hospitals received the bulk of their funding from public sources, they were more egalitarian in their admission standards than hospitals in the two other sectors, which had sources of funding that tended to serve specific groups. For-profit hospitals, which usually required patients to pay the full costs of service, were the most inegalitarian.

The sources and levels of funding of the three sectors tended to converge, however, particularly after the introduction of Medicare and Medicaid, causing the differences in their behavior to narrow. As investor-owned hospitals acquired greater access to capital markets and could fund much of their capital through reimbursement allowances, the differences in size and services between them and voluntary hospitals diminished. Similarly, investor-owned and nonprofit hospitals have increasingly received funds from the same third-

TABLE 1
Source of Funding, Ownership, and Behavior of Hospitals

	Public Hospitals Receiving Substantial Funding from the Public Sector	For-Profit Hospitals Receiving Substantial Funding from Paying Patients	Nonprofit Hospitals Receiving Substantial Funding from Philanthropy
Equality of access	+	−	−
Costs per client	−	−	+
Technological complexity	−	−	+
High-quality service	−	−	+
More personalized attention	−	+	+
Size	+	−	a

a. Larger than for-profit but smaller than public hospitals.

party payers, a tendency that has also narrowed the differences in their behavior. Small public hospitals of the same size as investor-owned and nonprofit hospitals have in recent years received more of their funding from similar sources, and their behavior has also converged with that of hospitals in the two other sectors.

The larger urban public hospitals, however, have continued to serve a disproportionate share of charity patients and to receive more funding per admission from local and state governments than hospitals in the other sectors. Hence, they have remained distinctly different, primarily because of the differences in funding and in the clients they serve.

Hospitals in all three sectors have been increasingly pressured into commercial orientation. These pressures, though strong in public hospitals, have been somewhat attenuated by the society-wide recognition that a high percentage of public hospitals are hospitals of last resort and that they cannot be expected to operate on the same basis as other hospitals. Voluntary and investor-owned hospitals have had much greater autonomy to interact with their environment. In contrast with the large urban public hospitals, most voluntary and investor-owned hospitals have been subject to somewhat different cost pressures and have therefore been able to respond differently. Increasing commercialism, built on the distinctive American system of fee for care, has begun to raise serious problems about the sense of mission of hospitals and particularly the care of the indigent. Hospitals in all three sectors face the problem of coping with the trade-off between budget pressures and the needs of the uninsured.

Despite the convergence in size, case mix, and sources of funding among hospitals in the three sectors, their behavior still varies. A historical perspective permits us to observe how the behavior of the sectors compares over time. The chapters that follow not only focus on that behavior but also try to explain the variation that persists both within and among the three sectors.

Notes

1. See Richard E. Caves, "Industrial Organization, Corporate Strategy and Structure," *Journal of Economic Literature*, vol. 18 (March 1980), pp. 64–92; Albert O. Hirschman, *Exit, Voice, and Loyalty* (Cambridge, Mass.: Harvard University Press, 1970); J. Rogers Hollingsworth, "The Snare of Specialization," *Bulletin of the Atomic Scientists*, vol. 40 (June/July 1984), pp. 34–37; Donald Pelz, "Creative Tensions in the Research and Development Climate," *Science*, vol. 157 (July 14, 1967), pp. 160–65; and Frank M. Andrews, *Scientific Productivity* (Cambridge: Cambridge University Press, 1979).

2. See Burton A. Weisbrod, *The Voluntary Non-Profit Sector* (Lexington, Mass.: Lexington Books, 1977); Marc Bendick, "Education as a Three-Sector Industry" (Ph.D. dissertation, University of Wisconsin, 1975); Mark Pauly and Michael Redisch, "The Not-for-Profit Hospital as a Physicians' Cooperative," *American Economic Review*, vol. 63 (1973), pp. 87–99; Henry B. Hansmann, "The Role of Nonprofit Enterprise," *Yale Law Journal*, vol. 89 (1980), pp. 835–901; Estelle James, "Production, Consumption and Cross-Subsidization in Non-Profit Organizations," Working Paper no. 30, Program on Non-Profit Organizations, Institution for Social and Policy Studies, Yale University; and Joseph P. Newhouse, "Toward a Theory of Nonprofit Institutions: An Economic Model of a Hospital," *American Economic Review*, vol. 60 (1970), pp. 64–74. The two most useful recent studies on nonprofit organizations in the health industry are Theodore R. Marmor, Mark Schlesinger, and Richard Smithey, "A New Look at Nonprofits: Health Care Policy in a Competitive Age," *Yale Journal of Regulation*, vol. 3 (Spring 1986), pp. 313–49; and Committee on Implications of For-Profit Enterprise in Health Care, Institute of Medicine, Bradford H. Gray, ed., *For-Profit Enterprise in Health Care* (Washington, D.C.: National Academy Press, 1986).

3. See the essays in E. S. Phelps, ed., *Altruism, Morality, and Economic Theory* (New York: Russell Sage Foundation, 1975), as well as the following: Kenneth J. Arrow, *Social Choice and Individual Values* (New Haven, Conn.: Yale University Press, 1963); and David Collard, *Altruism and Economy: A Study in Non-Selfish Economics* (Oxford: Martin Robertson, 1978).

4. Caves, "Industrial Organization"; Oliver Williamson, *Markets and Hierarchies: Analysis and Antitrust Implications* (New York: Free Press, 1975); Richard R. Nelson and Sidney G. Winters, *An Evolutionary Theory of Economic*

Change (Cambridge, Mass.: Harvard University Press, 1982); Lance E. Davis and D. C. North, *Institutional Change and American Economic Growth* (Cambridge: Cambridge University Press, 1971); Howard E. Aldrich, *Organizations and Environments* (Englewood Cliffs, N.J.: Prentice-Hall, 1979); John Freeman and Michael T. Hannan, "Growth and Decline Processes in Organizations," *American Sociological Review,* vol. 40 (April 1975), pp. 215–28; Michael Hannan and John Freeman, "The Population Ecology of Organizations," *American Journal of Sociology,* vol. 82 (March 1977), pp. 929–64; Paul R. Lawrence and Davis Dyer, *Renewing American Industry* (New York: Free Press, 1983); and Jeffrey Pfeffer and Gerald Salanick, *The External Control of Organizations: A Resource Dependence Perspective* (New York: Harper and Row, 1978).

5. Chris Argyris and Donald A. Shon, *Organizational Learning: A Theory of Action Perspective* (Reading, Mass.: Addison-Wesley, 1978); Lawrence and Dyer, *Renewing American Industry;* James March and Herbert Simon, *Organizations* (New York: John Wiley, 1958); and James March and Johan Olsen, *Ambiguity and Choice in Organizations* (Bergen, Norway: Unversitets Forlaget, 1976).

6. Alfred D. Chandler, Jr., *Strategy and Structure* (Cambridge, Mass.: MIT Press, 1962), and *The Visible Hand: The Managerial Revolution in American Business* (Cambridge, Mass.: Harvard University Press, 1977); and Rosemary Stevens, "The Changing Hospital," in Linda Aiken and David Mechanic, eds., *Applications of Social Science to Clinical Medicine Health Policy* (New Brunswick, N.J.: Rutgers University Press, 1986), pp. 80–99.

7. Kenneth Arrow, "Uncertainty and Medical Care," *American Economic Review,* vol. 53 (1963), pp. 941–73; Weisbrod, *Voluntary Non-Profit Sector;* and Julian LeGrand and Ray Robinson, *The Economics of Social Problems* (London: Macmillan, 1976).

8. For a theoretical discussion of these issues, see David B. Johnson, "The Fundamental Economics of the Charity Market" (Ph.D. dissertation, University of Virginia, 1968); Bruce Bolnick, "Toward a Behavioral Theory of Philanthropic Activity," in Phelps, *Altruism,* pp. 197–224; J. Rogers Hollingsworth, *A Political Economy of Medicine: Great Britain and the United States* (Baltimore: Johns Hopkins University Press, 1986); Peter Blau, *Exchange and Power in Social Life* (New York: John Wiley, 1984); and M. Mauss, *The Gift* (London: Cohen and West, 1966).

9. Stevens, "Changing Hospital"; and Donald W. Light, "Corporate Medicine for Profit," *Scientific American,* vol. 255 (December 1986), pp. 38–45.

10. The following is an interesting discussion of regulation in the hospital industry: Louise B. Russell, "Regulating the Diffusion of Hospital Technologies," *Law and Contemporary Problems,* vol. 43 (Winter-Spring 1979), pp. 26–42.

11. See the very interesting discussion in Jeff Charles Goldsmith, *Can Hospitals Survive?: The New Competitive Health Market* (Homewood, Ill.: Dow Jones–Irwin, 1981).

12. For a discussion of how technological complexity and the rate of technological change influence the size of firms, see J. Rogers Hollingsworth and Leon Lindberg, "The Governance of the American Economy: The Role of

Markets, Hierarchies, Clans, and Associations," in Wolfgang Streeck and Philippe C. Schmitter, ed., *Private Interest Government and Public Policy* (London and Beverly Hills: Sage Publications, 1985), pp. 221–54.

13. For a discussion of the "M-form" organizations, see Chandler, *Strategy and Structure* and *The Visible Hand;* Williamson, *Markets and Hierarchies;* and William G. Ouchi, *The M-Form Society* (Reading, Mass.: Addison-Wesley, 1984).

14. Richard W. Foster, "The Nonprofit Hospital: Evolution and Future Prospects" (Paper presented at the University of Chicago, September 1983).

15. On the history of vertical integration of American firms, see Chandler, *Strategy and Structure* and *The Visible Hand.* For economic theory on the vertical integration of firms and sectors, see Williamson, *Markets and Hierarchies,* pp. 82–131; and George J. Stigler, *The Organization of Industry* (Homewood, Ill.: Richard D. Irwin, 1968), pp. 129–41.

16. For support for this argument, see Hollingsworth, *Political Economy of Medicine;* and J. Rogers Hollingsworth and Ellen Jane Hollingsworth, "Differences between Voluntary and Public Organizations: The Behavior of Hospitals in England and Wales," *Journal of Health Politics, Policy and Law,* vol. 10 (Summer 1985), pp. 371–97.

2
The Development of the American Hospital Industry

This chapter is concerned with the circumstances under which acute-care or community hospitals came into being in the voluntary, public, and proprietary sectors and with the forces responsible for changes in the size and structure of the three sectors over a period of eighty years, from about 1900 to 1980. During the twentieth century the number of voluntary and public hospitals has grown markedly as the total number of general hospitals has increased. The number of hospitals in the proprietary sector, however, has substantially declined, although the number of beds in the proprietary sector has more than doubled since 1960 (see table 2). Much of the analysis is concerned with such variables as the availability and sources of capital and operating revenue, levels of technological complexity, and the relative homogeneity or heterogeneity of demand. The regulatory environment and the cultural expectations associated with general hospitals are also emphasized. These conditions have varied greatly in the twentieth century, as the services and facilities in general hospitals have changed and as the role of the federal government has been fundamentally altered.

Finally, the chapter addresses the rapid shifts in institutional arrangements of the past twenty years, as consolidation has taken place in the form of horizontal mergers and other multi-institutional arrangements. In recent years the extent to which hospitals have become associated with one another has considerably changed; so that now about one in three hospitals is affiliated in some way with another hospital.[1] Moreover, current literature has begun to stress how akin to other industries the hospital industry is—for example, in exhibiting greater concern with vertical and horizontal integration and in attempting to capitalize on economies of scale. These themes are explored in this chapter.

The discussion begins with voluntary hospitals, whose history illuminates the themes of community development and sectoral response set forth in chapter 1. In many ways the voluntary hospital is an exemplary indicator of the shifts in the twentieth-century American medical care system. After a discussion of voluntary hospitals, the analysis turns to public hospitals, then to proprietary hospitals, and finally to the major new multi-institutional arrangements that have arisen in the past twenty years.

Voluntary Hospitals

Origins. Voluntary hospitals have usually been considered the key to the American hospital system during the twentieth century. They were the quintessential acute-care hospitals only twenty-five years ago.[2] When *Modern Hospital* published extensive "prototype studies" of general hospitals during the 1950s, the data for the studies were all from voluntary hospitals. Throughout the twentieth century voluntary hospitals have had more beds than the hospitals in the two other sectors. As table 2 shows, in the past fifty-five years the number of voluntary hospitals has almost doubled and the number of beds more than tripled.

Because the origins of individual voluntary hospitals have been documented elsewhere in rich detail, here we indicate only the broad outlines of the institutionalization of the voluntary hospital sector in the eighteenth and nineteenth centuries. In many cities voluntary hospitals were created by interest groups or outstanding local leaders and businessmen who believed that some facility should be provided for the deserving poor and for travelers who had no place of succor when ill. Doctors were often active in promoting the establishment of a hospital. Sometimes founders had motives of religious obligation, viewing the founding of a hospital as an expression of their service to a higher being. Other hospitals originated to advance medical education and to serve special groups such as seamen, whose health problems in port cities required some response. In a few mountain states, the Western Federation of Miners established voluntary hospitals in the late nineteenth and early twentieth centuries to keep injured workers from being treated by company-controlled hospitals and physicians, who, it was feared, might minimize the seriousness of work-related injuries. At the same time in the South, philanthropists in large and small cities occasionally established hospitals for blacks, thus accommodating themselves to the realities of racial segregation. Regardless of the exact circumstances, voluntary hospitals were provided by the few for the few. Most citizens had no interest in creating hospitals and no intention of using them. Before the twentieth century the demand for general hospitals was small, although it was more widespread in large urban areas.[3]

TABLE 2

Nonfederal General and Short-Term Specialty Hospitals, 1909–1983
(beds in thousands)

Year	Government				Voluntary				For-Profit				Total	
	Hospitals	%	Beds	%	Hospitals	%	Beds	%	Hospitals	%	Beds	%	Hospitals	Beds
1909[a]									2,441	56			4,359	421
1925[a]													4,041	293
1928	540	12.5	81	24.1	1,889	43.9	197	58.6	1,877	43.6	58	17.3	4,306	336
1935	497	12.4	91	25.9	2,069	51.7	216	61.4	1,434	35.9	45	12.8	4,000	352
1940	568	13.6	120	30.0	2,338	56.1	242	60.5	1,259	30.2	38	9.5	4,165	400
1946	785	17.7	133	28.1	2,584	58.1	301	63.6	1,076	24.2	39	8.2	4,445	473
1950	942	18.7	131	25.9	2,871	57.1	332	65.7	1,218	24.2	42	8.3	5,031	505
1955	1,120	21.4	142	25.0	3,097	59.1	389	68.5	1,020	19.5	37	6.5	5,237	568
1960	1,260	23.3	156	24.4	3,291	60.9	446	69.8	856	15.8	37	5.8	5,407	639

1965	1,453	25.3	179	24.2	3,426	59.7	515	69.5	857	14.9	47	6.3	5,736	741
1970	1,704	29.1	204	24.0	3,386	57.8	592	69.7	769	13.1	53	6.2	5,859	849
1975	1,840	30.8	215	22.7	3,364	56.3	659	69.6	775	13.0	73	7.7	5,979	947
1980	1,835	31.1	212	21.4	3,339	56.6	693	69.9	730	12.4	87	8.8	5,904	992
1983	1,723	29.5	209	20.5	3,363	57.6	718	70.3	757	13.0	94	9.2	5,843	1,021

a. 1909 and 1925 data include all types of hospitals.

SOURCES: 1909: Bureau of the Census, *Historical Statistics of the United States*, pt. 1 (Washington, D.C., 1975), p. 78. The proprietary hospital data are estimates. See Bruce Steinwald and Duncan Neuhauser, "The Role of the Proprietary Hospital," *Journal of Law and Contemporary Problems*, vol. 35 (1970), pp. 818–19. 1925: "Hospital Service in the United States," *Journal of the American Medical Association*, vol. 86, no. 14 (April 3, 1926), p. 1009. Data include federal general hospitals. 1928: C. Rufus Rorem, *The Public's Investment in Hospitals* (Chicago: University of Chicago Press, 1930), p. 14. 1935: "Hospital Service in the United States," *Journal of the American Medical Association*, vol. 106, no. 10 (March 7, 1936), p. 792. 1940: "Hospital Service in the United States," *Journal of the American Medical Association*, vol. 116, no. 11 (March 15, 1941), p. 1057. Control of 2,000 beds not given. 1946–1955: *Guide to the Health Care Field* (Chicago: American Hospital Association, 1976), pp. 7–9. 1960–1983: *Statistical Abstract of the United States 1985*, p. 106.

During much of the nineteenth century voluntary hospitals were governed primarily by the private philanthropists who created and financed them. Private rather than public money provided the capital for acquiring and improving hospitals and made up almost the whole of their operating budgets, and most patients received free services. Because voluntary hospitals were providing community services, however, state and local governments sometimes made contributions for their establishment. The Massachusetts legislature provided a small subsidy to assist in establishing the Massachusetts General Hospital, the Pennsylvania Hospital received a grant from the Provincial Assembly, and the city of Milwaukee provided land for a Catholic hospital in the 1850s.

The medical staff was chosen by trustees of the hospital, who also made the decisions about the kinds of cases suitable for admission. Persons who were contagious, vagrant, or morally suspect were not welcome in most voluntary hospitals. The mentally ill and chronically ill were also not admitted. Rather, most voluntary hospitals were for the "deserving poor," the citizens who could not recover in their usual residences (servants in fashionable homes, for example). In the nineteenth century hospitals provided not only medical care but also shelter and food for those in need. Their paternalism carried implications for the conduct of both patients and staff.[4]

At the time the earliest voluntary hospitals were established in the United States, the hospital was primarily custodial; it could offer little in the way of cure. The risk of infection was so great and the mortality from surgery so high that hospitals were used only as a last resort by most patients. Middle- and upper-income groups who could summon medical care to come to them made virtually no use of hospitals. They preferred to be treated at home, even to have surgery at home.

After the Civil War conditions in hospitals slowly changed with the advancement of knowledge about the relation between sanitation and infection. Surgical techniques improved, and with the discovery of anesthesia, surgery became less risky and more common.[5] As a result of these changes, the hospital became involved in active treatment of cases.

Still, as late as 1870 there were relatively few hospitals. Joseph Toner of the U.S. Bureau of Education estimated that in 1873 there were only 178 hospitals in the United States, and one-third of those were mental hospitals. Many hospitals were in the nation's largest cities, where commercial travelers needed them in case of accident or illness.[6]

Social and economic conditions in the late nineteenth and early twentieth centuries gave rise to a dramatic upsurge of hospital construction, mainly in the voluntary sector. Underlying this expansion of general hospitals were several factors: (1) greater popular belief in medical efficacy, which increased the demand for hospital care; (2) changes in demographic patterns, which moved the treatment of illness from the home to the hospital; (3) increased population heterogeneity as a result of immigration; and (4) greater availability of capital for hospital construction. Some of these factors led to an increase in the number of all kinds of general hospitals, not just voluntary hospitals. The increased belief in medical efficacy and increased demand for hospitals, for example, were related to the founding of hospitals in all three sectors, whereas population heterogeneity and the availability of philanthropic capital were more closely linked to the number of voluntary hospitals.[7]

One force that led to the creation of hundreds of hospitals was the change in medical technology during the last half of the nineteenth century. Scientific findings about the spread and origin of disease and about the means of controlling it, coupled with antisepsis and later asepsis for surgical procedures, gave the medical profession and hospitals new roles. According to Rosemary Stevens, by the early part of the twentieth century "surgery became enormously fashionable, and the American hospitals developed largely on the ethic and ethos of surgery."[8]

Irrespective of whether medical technology was actually efficacious, doctors and hospitals enjoyed enhanced legitimacy. Increasingly, people believed that doctors and hospitals provided the means for better health. More and more Americans no longer viewed entry to the hospital merely as a step on the way to the morgue but began to see the hospital as a place in which discomfort could be relieved. Thus after 1900 hospitals became more attractive to middle- and upper-income groups. In most voluntary hospitals the average length of stay declined with the rise in the percentage of patients having surgery.

The rapid urbanization of American society was also important in expanding the number of hospitals. Swollen by streams of immigrants and former rural residents, cities were places into which ever more people were crowded. Work accidents became more common as a result of employment in factories, and in very crowded living spaces recuperation at home was difficult at best. There was no extra room for a convalescent patient and often no one at home to provide nursing or company. The hospital thus became an alternative place in which the suffering patient might have rest, space, and some medical supervision and intervention.[9]

These factors—belief in increased efficacy and increased need due to urban conditions—underlay hospital expansion in all three sectors. Expansion in the voluntary sector, however, was uniquely fueled by two other important factors: the ethnic and religious heterogeneity of the population and the availability of philanthropic capital. These were closely intertwined, since the minorities usually mobilized the capital. Overall, though, it was the cultural heterogeneity of American society that, more than any other factor, was responsible for the emergence of the voluntary sector on a scale greater than in most other societies.

By the late nineteenth century many areas of the United States had quite heterogeneous populations because of diverse sources of immigration. Most immigrant groups maintained a distinct social identity in the United States or at least attempted to do so. They often had their own voluntary organizations, many of which were able to raise capital for services that would promote the group's goals. They founded churches, published newspapers in familiar languages, and often founded their own hospitals and schools. The older the community and the more prosperous and cohesive the immigrant ethnic or religious minority, the greater the probability that the group would use some of its wealth to create hospitals or would mobilize donations from others.

Immigrant groups often found that existing hospitals were cold and unfriendly places in which their native languages were not spoken or understood. Immigrant doctors were often not recognized, and immigrant patients had difficulty in receiving medical services from "their own people." The increasing pluralism of the American population, especially in the large urban areas where industrialism had wrought the greatest changes, led to the creation of many new voluntary hospitals to serve such special populations. Hospitals often took the names of the ethnic groups. There could be no question that the German Hospital was mainly for Germans or the Dublin Hospital for the Irish. If hospitals oriented their care toward particular ethnic groups, it was more likely that immigrant doctors could receive staff appointments and that immigrant patients would not be treated like outcasts because of their ethnic background or language.[10]

Many voluntary hospitals, which often had only a few beds, were located in ethnic enclaves, very accessible to the local population. Unlike earlier philanthropic hospitals, they were often created by people who thought they might personally use them. Some religious- or ethnic-based hospitals made it a firm policy that patients of all backgrounds would be admitted and did not focus exclusively on "their own."[11] Others made much less of a point of their general availability. Early voluntary hospitals had served all the "deserving" destitute of a particular community, but by the end of the nineteenth century, many of the newer ethnic hospitals restricted their admissions primarily to the groups that founded them.

Ethnicity was only one of several factors associated with the creation of new voluntary hospitals. Religious pluralism was another. By 1928 church-sponsored hospitals throughout the country numbered 841, with over 100,000 beds. Although church-sponsored voluntary hospitals were outnumbered by other voluntary hospitals, church hospitals provided more beds and had more capital investment than independent hospitals.[12]

Orders of Catholic sisters were famous throughout the country for founding and administering hospitals. Some of these hospitals were both religiously and ethnically based, and some were founded to serve the whole community rather than special groups. The era of the founding of Catholic hospitals began about 1840. This was not simply a phenomenon that occurred in large cities; it was also very common for smaller communities with sizable Catholic populations to urge Catholic sisters to open a local hospital. The Catholic order need not contribute all the capital, but local leaders believed that church assistance would provide both legitimacy and nursing services to the new venture. Catholic hospitals almost always bore religious names, such as Mercy, St. Mary's, St. Joseph's, or Misericordia.[13]

Protestant groups, too, created hospitals. Presbyterians, Methodists, Baptists, and Lutherans were especially prominent in the establishment of hospitals in the Middle West. In some instances religious hospitals added acute-care facilities to sanitariums they had founded. In a number of large cities Jewish philanthropists also became involved in establishing hospitals, partly to provide a place in which Jewish physicians could practice but also to express religious convictions about responsibility by serving Jewish patients.[14]

There were also voluntary hospitals for blacks. After the Civil War both federal and private black hospitals were founded in southern and northern cities. Although many did not survive, others benefited from private philanthropic support and were able to remain open after support from public authorities ceased. Since most voluntary and public hospitals admitted only whites or had segregated wings and staffs, there were strong pressures to maintain separate, private black hospitals.[15]

Another important factor in the expansion of the voluntary hospital sector was the availability of philanthropic capital. If all citizens had preferred the same kind of hospital with equal intensity, no doubt the public sector would have attempted to satisfy that demand.

25

This was certainly not the case, however; many religious and ethnic groups demanded hospitals of their own. But the demand by various minorities for different kinds of hospitals could be met only if there were sufficient capital. Ethnic and religious groups canvassed their own members and buttonholed the wealthy, providing their own energy to mobilize capital for hospitals. Usually, the more cohesive the ethnic or religious group, the greater its ability to raise capital. When there was frequent and intense communication within ethnic and religious groups, it was more likely that funds could be obtained. Since almost all funding came from local sources, control of the hospitals remained local. To maintain financial support, hospitals found it necessary to be responsive to local demands.

Because voluntary hospitals depended on their communities for philanthropic support, they became increasingly oriented to serving those communities. Operating in a world before public welfare services were highly institutionalized, those who managed voluntary hospitals were often imbued with a mission and a spirit of serving public needs. Since voluntary hospitals served the needs of the community, local and state governments gave them special privileges and exemptions. In the late 1870s, for example, the courts ruled that because the Massachusetts General Hospital was a public charity, it could not be held liable for damages to its patients.[16] The expectation of stewardship from voluntary hospitals led to special tax incentives, which still endure. As long as a voluntary hospital provided free care, it was seen as an institution serving the community and one that in return deserved the financial, moral, and political support of the community.

Regional differences in wealth and population heterogeneity created regional variations in the availability of philanthropic capital and in the development of voluntary hospitals in the late nineteenth and early twentieth centuries.[17] In the Northeast, with a rich variety of immigrant groups, well-organized denominations, and established communities, the means existed to solicit and mobilize capital for hospital construction in the voluntary sector. In the middle Atlantic and middle western states, too, the considerable cultural pluralism was instrumental in providing the organizational means of mobilizing philanthropic capital. In some communities local capitalists were willing to make substantial donations to voluntary hospitals. Their motives were mixed: some saw such donations as appropriate to their stewardship of riches; others sought to keep workers healthy and productive through timely medical intervention; and still others were seeking to enhance their legitimacy as good citizens.[18] Throughout the northeastern, middle Atlantic, and middle western states in the years from 1890 to 1920, voluntary hospitals were founded in most communities with over 15,000 residents.

Relatively few voluntary hospitals were created in less wealthy or newer regions such as the Far West and the Deep South. In the western states population density was insufficient to create the demand for a hospital. Moreover, local elites often had very new wealth and were uninterested in community responsibility. Towns were too new and raw for civic consciousness to be strong, and in many communities religious and ethnic organizations were not powerful enough to create hospitals.

The southeastern states also had few hospitals for their population. The South traditionally had a shortage of capital, and its lack of urbanization made locating hospitals to serve patients difficult. With a sizable percentage of the population handicapped by poverty and racial discrimination, the financial base for voluntary hospitals was slim. Moreover, the largest southern minority—the blacks—did not have the financial resources to create hospitals.

Persistence of the Voluntary Sector and Changes in the Source of Operating Revenues. During the twentieth century the number of voluntary hospitals increased steadily until very recently. From 1928 to 1950 the number grew by approximately 10 percent per decade, although growth was somewhat slowed by the economic hardships of the depression. The number of voluntary hospital beds rose even more rapidly.

The reasons for the persistence and expansion of the voluntary sector are complex, of course. Many of the explanations for the origins of voluntary hospitals apply as well to their persistence. The ethnic and religious pluralism of American society meant that many hospitals in large cities were tied to well-organized groups that continued to support them. Many groups continued to provide philanthropic support for capital expansion of hospitals. Moreover, the large sunk costs contributed to the hospitals' continued operation, especially when buildings had been expensive. Paul Starr has suggested that many nonprofit hospitals persisted because the ethnic and religious groups associated with their founding were disinclined to merger or closure. Such groups were concerned that the people they wanted to protect ("their clientele") would be disregarded unless their hospitals continued to operate.[19] Since voluntary hospitals had vague and imprecise goals, there was no clear standard for deciding when to close them. Because they were more dependent on narrow interest groups than on large public authorities, voluntary hospitals, particularly in urban areas, were small and numerous. Their large number made for a somewhat uneconomical and inefficient hospital system.

The key factor in the survival of voluntary hospitals was their ability to obtain new sources of capital as well as revenues for daily operations, to move away from their early dependence on charity. Of course, the extent to which they had been charitable institutions is a complicated story. Rosemary Stevens has written that "voluntary hospitals were never really charities."[20] In the nineteenth century patients had generally been expected to pay hospital board if they could afford to do so, although physicians who practiced in many hospitals did so gratuitously. Traditionally, most voluntary hospitals refrained from charging any significant amount for their services because it was assumed that patients were too poor to pay for care. And because the costs of operation were relatively low, a few wealthy benefactors could generally guarantee the solvency of a hospital.[21]

During the 1890s, however, the financial condition of voluntary hospitals began to change. Technological change raised the costs of operation, and the economic depression of the 1890s substantially increased the number of people making demands on voluntary hospitals. As a result, philanthropists could no longer provide enough donations to cover the deficits that the hospitals were experiencing. By the turn of the century, charity was proving an inadequate means of supporting hospitals, which soon recognized that their traditional role of serving the "deserving poor," with philanthropists paying most of the bill, was outmoded. They began to turn their attention to middle-income patients who could pay for their care. Brooklyn Hospital, for example, received only 12 percent of its revenues from paying patients in 1892 but 61 percent by 1905. Many trustees of voluntary hospitals began to be contemptuous of patients who could not afford to pay.[22]

Of course, sources of income varied, but all across the country voluntary hospitals were becoming more dependent on paying patients. We must not exaggerate, however, the extent of their dependence. A 1904 national census of hospitals found that voluntary hospitals received 54.4 percent of their operating revenues from paying patients and 9.5 percent from government subsidies. The rest—36.1 percent—came primarily from contributions and endowments.[23]

Voluntary hospitals were able to prosper and persist by changing their character in the twentieth century. As medical technology became more complex and expensive, they changed from primarily custodial to treatment centers, from caring for mostly poor to treating mostly middle-income patients. As their clientele changed, their management became increasingly entrepreneurial. Slowly they began to resemble hotels more than almshouses, while their earlier paternalism became more business oriented. To bring in paying patients, voluntary hospitals—especially large ones—began to place more emphasis on good food, pleasant accommodations, and other amenities.

Along with increased dependence on paying patients came greater reliance on business-oriented trustees. Financial solvency required good business management and steady, sizable flows of patients rather than the former emphasis on paternalism. To be sure of an adequate supply of patients, hospitals awarded hospital privileges to more doctors. They were particularly generous in awarding privileges to surgeons.

For doctors, the voluntary hospital tended to become an adjunct of their private practice; as this occurred, their gratuitous provision of services for most of their hospital patients became a thing of the past. This was in contrast to Europe, where hospital-based doctors more and more became employees of hospitals.

Although the public purse provided only 9.5 percent of the income of voluntary hospitals at the turn of the century, a few city governments were paying a per diem amount for treating patients on a means-tested basis. A precedent had been established on which the society would build in the 1960s with the inauguration of the Medicaid program: state authorities would certify that certain classes of indigent patients were eligible to receive care, and the state would reimburse the hospital.[24]

During the 1920s and 1930s voluntary hospitals obtained small amounts of public funding in other ways, primarily as reimbursement for caring for the poor. For example, during the 1930s many voluntary hospitals in large urban areas obtained public reimbursement for outpatient services for the poor. This use of tax funds was not nearly so extensive as subsidies for inpatient care, but it did occur, principally in communities with limited outpatient services in public hospitals.[25]

Another factor associated with the persisting strength of the voluntary hospital sector was the slowness of public authorities to assume widespread responsibility for hospital services. Partly because public services were historically restricted primarily to those in most extreme need or to services that were homogeneously demanded, there was little public initiative in the delivery of acute hospital services until well into the twentieth century. As a result most American communities before the Second World War provided a narrow range of public services and relied on tax revenues no more than was absolutely necessary.

Until the 1960s many voluntary hospitals successfully continued to raise money from philanthropic sources. The continued dependence on the community for support led to the persistence of a particular ethos among voluntary hospitals—to the belief that even if most patients paid for their care, the voluntary hospital had an obligation to serve the community and to carry out a mission of good will. In the twentieth century, however, donations have usually been for specified purposes. Rich families and individuals have attempted to endow a specific facility in a voluntary hospital, frequently named after a particular individual. Giving to the hospital's general endowment or operating budget has become less frequent.[26]

Between the two world wars, further shifts occurred in the authority structure of voluntary hospitals, as the medical staff gained even greater importance in the making of decisions. The doctors, who sent the patients to the hospitals and decided what treatment was appropriate, became paramount in deciding about buying equipment, expanding beds and facilities, raising capital for plant modification, and the like. Surgeons, as controllers of very important technology, became particularly significant in shaping hospital decisions. The voluntary hospital had become a community-funded workshop for the doctor—a place in which he could carry out his professional activities without being financially at risk. He and his colleagues decided what features the workshop should have, and medical administrators were on hand to carry out their wishes.

By the end of the Second World War, American voluntary hospitals had moved quite far from their original client bases. As technology became more expensive and more people demanded access to hospitals, an increasingly small percentage of patients were free or charity cases. Voluntary hospitals increasingly relied on complex systems of medical insurance, beginning with workmen's compensation in the early part of the century. By the 1940s and 1950s hospital insurance had become widespread, so that the sources of operating revenues were varied. By the late 1950s some form of insurance payment was made for almost 74 percent of voluntary hospital patients, and in over half the discharges from voluntary hospitals, the insurer paid more than three-fourths of the bill. The rising costs for more and more complex technology required that patients have some regular financial arrangements for meeting hospital bills. Neither philanthropy nor out-of-pocket payments were adequate for large bills. Insurance not only reassured the patient but also provided a more secure base for hospitals.[27]

Without the spread of private insurance the future of voluntary hospitals would have been severely threatened. For all practical purposes, hospital insurance in America began with Blue Cross plans during the depression of the 1930s. Because many patients were unable to pay their bills and many hospitals were experiencing financial difficulties, the voluntary hospital sector responded by helping to develop hospital insurance, which helped keep them solvent. In many instances hospitals agreed to share risk with Blue Cross plans; if payouts exceeded income, hospitals would share in the loss. Because voluntary hospitals had firmly established their community role by 1920, their legitimacy extended to the new Blue Cross plans, which were usually sponsored by voluntary hospitals. Meanwhile ties between the Blue Cross plans and the American Hospital Association (AHA) were very strong; the AHA took a decisive lead in setting forth the characteristics for Blue Cross plans, especially the importance of hospital representation on Blue Cross boards.

The distinctive features of Blue Cross plans were as follows:

• They were service plans that paid the hospital for specific services rather than indemnity plans that paid cash amounts to the covered consumer.

• They provided community experience ratings, so that everyone in a community could join at roughly the same rate. This kind of rating made hospital insurance available to low-income persons and small groups at costs lower than they would otherwise have been. This effectively subsidized insurance for poor and elderly persons who could afford medical insurance and had high medical expenses.

• Free choice of hospitals was open to all who enrolled. Because Blue Cross plans negotiated lower reimbursement rates for voluntary than for proprietary hospitals, they helped to accelerate the decline in the number of proprietary hospitals.

• The plans were to be nonprofit, with no one permitted to share any profits they might acquire.

• Most plans paid only for hospital care and not for physicians' services.

The founders of Blue Cross insurance plans wanted to differentiate their activities from commercial insurance companies. They did this by employing the ideals of community service and their nonprofit status.[28]

As Blue Cross plans became more numerous and competition with commercial insurers more explicit, Blue Cross organizations began to move away from community ratings. But because Blue Cross initially billed itself as providing a service to the community through affordable participation, it could secure special privileges from state and federal governments. In many states Blue Cross plans were granted exemption from the incorporation and reserve requirements imposed on commercial insurance companies and from paying property taxes as well as taxes on earned income. This preferential treatment remained long after the community service role became smaller.

The role of Blue Cross has varied over time and from region to region. In the eastern United States, voluntary hospitals and Blue Cross plans have been strongly intertwined. The plans have usually covered a very sizable fraction of the population, and they have been more likely to preserve community ratings and thereby to provide greater access for individuals and small groups with modest resources. In the mid-1970s Blue Cross covered almost 80 percent of the population in parts of New England, where voluntary hospitals were strong, but only 15 percent in southern California, where the for-profit hospital sector was vigorous. By 1969 some 35 percent of people under sixty-five carried hospital insurance with Blue Cross, and in 1985 a total of 80 million Americans were Blue Cross subscribers. Moreover, Blue Cross organizations became the fiscal intermediaries for a high proportion of persons covered by Medicare, another indication of how closely integrated Blue Cross was with the hospital industry.[29]

Blue Cross helped voluntary hospitals to survive, to maintain their fiscal integrity, and to remain autonomous. Reimbursed for a large fraction of charges by Blue Cross organizations in which they played an important role, the hospitals could usually be confident that their organizational preferences would be honored. Although in its early days Blue Cross had been a plan for individuals and small groups, it became increasingly a plan for large groups, in which the employer—not the employee—paid. Neither consumer nor hospital had any incentive to worry greatly about costs. To compete with commercial insurers and to win group contracts, Blue Cross usually bargained with hospitals to secure lower rates, but even so over the longer term it served to fuel hospital expansion and cost inflation, not to contain them.

At the same time Blue Cross plans, like the voluntary hospitals with which they were integrated, sought to differentiate themselves from for-profit organizations. Even as they began to behave very much like commercial insurance companies—particularly on the West Coast—they sought to convince the public that they were very different. For political reasons Blue Cross executives consciously used such terms as members instead of policy holders, rates instead of premiums, service instead of indemnity, enrolling instead of selling, and enrollment representatives instead of salesmen. All in all, Blue Cross organizations have sought, like voluntary hospitals, to maintain a reputation as public interest organizations serving the good of the communities in which they operate and therefore deserving of preferential treatment from the state. Their success in maintaining this reputation has helped them to survive. More important, Blue Cross plans have been able to survive because they have increasingly tried to offer the same kinds of policies as the commercial insurers— that is, policies based on the experience of particular groups rather than community rating. Thus for at least two decades most Blue Cross plans have eliminated the implicit subsidy to high-risk persons.[30]

Changes in the Source of Capital: The Role of the Federal Government. By 1940 the voluntary hospital system was extremely well entrenched in American society, made up largely of hospitals that had originally come into existence in response to minorities dissatisfied with public provision of facilities. As long as dissatisfied groups could mobilize capital, often through ethnic or religious appeals, they could create voluntary hospitals. Many small towns and rural areas, however, had insufficient wealth to support either a public or a voluntary nonprofit hospital. In 1946, responding to the presence of many underserved areas, Congress created the Hill-Burton program, which made it possible for many smaller communities to establish hospitals, often voluntary hospitals.

From the viewpoint of the federal government, the purpose of Hill-Burton was threefold: (1) to assist states in conducting an inventory and needs assessment of medical facilities; (2) to provide part of the funding for the construction of hospitals; and (3) to stimulate local capital, which was required to match the 30 percent federal contribution. Funds were made available under the Hill-Burton program for both new construction and renovation of existing facilities. Public and voluntary organizations might benefit from Hill-Burton, but proprietary organizations were excluded. Because the voluntary sector contained about 60 percent of all general hospitals and beds and was the prototype for acute care, it was inconceivable to Congress that it be excluded from Hill-Burton funding. Its unquestioned legitimacy gave it access to public money.

Hill-Burton funding was allocated to states according to their per capita income and health needs—the states that were most "underbedded" received the largest sums of money, and those with the most beds for their population received proportionately smaller sums. The legislation was intended not simply to provide beds but to provide them in areas of acute shortage.

Significantly, the American medical profession had historically been hostile to the idea of federally funded medical insurance, for fear it would lead to state interference with the doctor-patient relationship. Federal funding of hospital construction, however, was an entirely different matter, which doctors saw as no threat to the doctor-patient relationship. More important, doctors needed the hospital to carry out their professional responsibilities, and many were unwilling to locate in a community that lacked a local hospital.

During the period when it funded hospital construction (1946–1973), the Hill-Burton program was modified several times. In the early years of the program most Hill-Burton funds were used to provide general hospital beds in small cities, towns, or rural areas. Among projects for new facilities, the emphasis on small communities was very strong, particularly in southern states. About 44 percent of the inpatient beds were in communities outside standard metropolitan statistical areas, and about 57 percent of the new general hospital projects by 1963 provided fewer than fifty beds. Over time, however, Hill-Burton funding was used more and more to renovate existing facilities, urban hospitals, and facilities for long-term care. The Hill-Burton program—still in operation—requires many hospitals to provide a specified amount of indigent care in return for federal money. Without this provision many voluntary hospitals would probably provide less indigent care than they do today.[31]

The significance of Hill-Burton was that the federal government was contributing to construction and expansion of voluntary hospitals and to their purchase of medical equipment rather than directing its resources exclusively to public authorities. During the years of Hill-Burton, the number of general voluntary hospitals increased by approximately 30 percent and the number of general hospital beds by approximately 119 percent.

Hill-Burton funds contributed not only to the persistence of the voluntary sector but also to its expansion. Areas previously without adequate capital found that with federal assistance they could afford voluntary hospitals. Nevertheless, the complex rules for obtaining Hill-Burton funds have occasionally been interpreted as favoring communities that already had hospitals and wanted to use the funds to expand them. It is true that communities without hospitals and without specialists in hospital management generally lacked the skill necessary to comply with federal planning requirements and frequently experienced difficulty in obtaining Hill-Burton funds. Most Hill-Burton funding, however, was used for small community hospitals. The federal government, by helping to expand hospital capacity, was contributing to improved access to medical care.[32]

New Sources of Revenue and Dependence. The next important development affecting the financing of the hospital sector was the enactment of the Medicare and Medicaid programs in 1965. These were designed to provide third-party medical coverage for millions of elderly and low-income Americans who had usually been without such coverage. Not only were the rules for Medicare and Medicaid coverage and reimbursement very complicated, but, with many private payment schemes, the entire system of hospital financing became extraordinarily complex.

Medicare was essentially a federal entitlement program covering a specific age group and a much smaller number of disabled persons, with standardized nonstigmatizing features. Although it did not relieve participants of all liability for costs, it created virtually no intervention between provider and client, leaving to clients the choice of doctor and hospital. By 1981 Medicare was the source of approximately one-third of the revenue of general hospitals.[33]

Medicaid was quite different, with much more variation among states. Designed for the poor, Medicaid programs were funded by federal, state, and local authorities, but conditions of entitlement and benefits were set mostly by the states. Only a relatively small fraction of Medicaid expenses were for inpatient care in community hospitals, and a relatively small percentage of patients in most voluntary hospitals had their bills paid by Medicaid.

With the inauguration of Medicare, hospitals were presented with a sizable population of patients whose bills were substantially guaranteed. A minority of these patients had been covered by third-party payment plans, but Medicare provided patients, doctors, and hospitals with substantial financial gain. Hospitals were able to create facilities and supply services for many new clients. Both Medicare and Medicaid usually reimbursed hospitals at higher rates than states had used for those on public assistance. Before 1965 states had negotiated with both voluntary and public hospitals for rates well below costs.

Although the American Hospital Association had vigorously opposed federal medical insurance, the financial rewards from Medicare and Medicaid were almost instantly recognized. Medicare permitted depreciation to be included in calculating the costs of serving patients, including depreciation of Hill-Burton assets. That provision reimbursed hospitals more for newer and usually more expensive facilities. Neither Medicare nor Medicaid, however, would allow hospitals to include the costs of charity in calculating reimbursement costs for covered beneficiaries.

The price of medical services, subject to minor inflation before the Medicare and Medicaid programs, grew dramatically after their passage. Indeed, the expansion of private medical insurance, along with Medicare and Medicaid, was a major factor in the rapid growth of hospital costs. With a retrospective form of third-party payment and

35

few deductibles to be paid by the patient, doctors, hospitals, and patients had few incentives to economize on costs.[34]

The effect of Medicare was considerable not only among voluntary hospitals but also among public and proprietary hospitals. In all three sectors hospitals saw Medicare as an opportunity to expand their beds and facilities. Many voluntary hospitals believed that their services would be better if their facilities were more elaborate and if they acquired more beds. All hospitals could pass a substantial portion of the costs of new and expensive technology to the federal government. Specialized facilities were thought to be attractive to doctors admitting clients, and more admissions would mean more business for such facilities. These anticipations relied on circular reasoning, but the bottom line was the expansion of capital equipment.

Between 1965 and 1975 third-party payers—both governmental and private—lavished resources on the hospital sector. Hospital costs grew much more rapidly than the consumer price index. The number of hospital beds expanded substantially in each sector, and most hospitals attempted to acquire the latest medical technology. As hospitals expanded and turned their attention to extracting from third-party payers the maximum reimbursement for treatment, the authority structure within hospitals underwent another shift.

Many hospitals turned to professional managers or administrators, rather than continuing to rely on the medical staff. Such a change was also a response to the increasing differentiation of structures within hospitals, which had its roots in the advances that had taken place in medical care. As hospitals became more differentiated internally, they needed managers skilled in the art of negotiating differences among competing parts of complex organizations. In some instances, of course, doctor-administrators, with their staffs of experts, continued to dominate voluntary hospitals, interacting with the medical staff with varying degrees of tension. The more common pattern, however, was for professional administrators, skilled in dealing with third-party payers, to take over many of the chores of running a hospital while giving careful deference to the doctors who brought patients into the hospital. The differentiation of medical services also led to differentiation in administrative tasks, so that it became commonplace for large hospitals to have large, professional administrative staffs.[35]

With the coming of Medicare, the voluntary hospitals departed further from certain basic traditions. Historically they had assumed multiple roles in American communities as providers of medical services, insurance agencies, and welfare organizations. Since the introduction of Medicare, they have been much less involved in insurance

36

and welfare. Earlier, many voluntary hospitals acted as insurance organizations for religious and ethnic groups, in that donors were motivated to give money to ensure that they and their fellow citizens would have a hospital available if they became ill. Once Blue Cross, commercial insurance organizations, and Medicare became third-party payers, the insurance functions of the voluntary hospital declined.

By providing charity to those in need, the voluntary hospital had long assumed the functions of a welfare organization. Medicare and Medicaid, by paying the costs of care for the elderly and the poor, reduced the charitable role of the hospital. Once public authorities were assuming fiscal responsibility, voluntary hospitals could make less of a case for philanthropic giving. Nor did they need philanthropy to the same extent. As a proportion of total income, philanthropic giving to voluntary hospitals peaked in 1964–1965. By 1981 philanthropic contributions to hospitals as a percentage of personal income had dropped to the lowest level since 1929, less than one-fourth of the level when Medicare began.[36]

Under Medicare hospitals were reimbursed for interest expenses incurred for debt, as well as for depreciation. Because of the reimbursement formula, hospitals in all three sectors increasingly resorted to debt to finance capital equipment. Thus local hospital administrators since the mid-1960s have devoted less energy to local fund raising. Recent changes in the federal tax code have further reduced the incentive to make donations to voluntary hospitals. Once the very existence of such hospitals was based on local giving, but after the mid-1960s third-party payment schemes diminished the community's fund-raising efforts. Each hospital increasingly competed for its share of the federal pie, with less concern for local accountability.[37]

Not only have the sources of capital and operating revenues for voluntary hospitals changed, but in large cities their religious and ethnic ties have been weakened. As ethnic consciousness diminished and as white middle- and upper-income groups moved in large numbers from central cities to suburban communities, many voluntary hospitals lost the allegiance of the groups that had spawned their development and became increasingly dependent on third-party payers for their survival. As local hospitals, rigidly tied to a specific location, many were trapped in a kind of limbo.

External Efforts to Control Costs. Before the late 1960s the medical policies of the federal government had given high priority to providing American citizens with greater access to medical care, by funding the cost of hospital construction and by removing barriers that impeded access by the poor and the elderly. Cost considerations were given relatively low priority. As hospitals expanded and costs soared, however, the federal and state governments eventually reversed priorities and tried to contain hospital spending. The rules for Medicare reimbursement were eventually so dramatically altered that some hospitals began to complain that they actually lost money by treating Medicare patients. In 1983 Frank Sloan wrote that "Medicare has become a relatively 'frugal' or 'tight' payer . . . even in a world of retrospective reimbursement." In 1981 Medicare was reimbursing hospitals in Colorado at approximately 20 percent below what other payers were reimbursing for the same services.[38]

The federal and state governments adopted a variety of regulatory strategies in an effort to control hospital spending. The most important were more rational planning of resource distribution, rate setting, and decisions about admissions and use.

The most visible aspect of early regulatory programs was the certificate-of-need (CON) program, which required hospitals to obtain prior approval from a state agency before engaging in certain kinds of capital expansion. By 1979 forty-nine states had CON programs. The better evaluation studies have concluded that CON controls had little effect on per capita expenditures for hospital services, although they did affect the composition of services. CON programs altered the rate of bed growth in some hospitals but not in others. Moreover, they did little to control the purchase of expensive equipment by private parties, which leased it to hospitals.[39]

Another dimension of regulation was utilization review, enacted in the early 1970s in the guise of professional services review organizations (PSROs). Focused on the examination of medical records of beneficiaries of federal insurance programs, PSROs depended on professionals' setting and enforcing standards of appropriate care for patients. While the evidence on the effects of the program is mixed, PSRO programs may have contributed slightly to shortening average hospital stays, without lowering per capita use of hospitals or eliminating unnecessary costs.[40]

A third major regulatory strategy employed in the 1970s was review of the rates that hospitals charged to patients. Such review was undertaken primarily by the states and was intended to prevent further escalation of costs. State programs varied in the extent to which they were mandatory or voluntary and whether they applied to most or to all payers. Recent analysis of the effects of these programs has suggested that they had a negligible effect in their early years but became slightly more effective after three years and that only mandatory programs had any effect on costs. States in which all payers were subject to rate review were better able than other states to achieve results. Evaluations of these programs are complicated, and the results should be treated with caution.[41]

The ballooning costs of Medicare and the impending inadequacies of the Medicare trust funds led the federal government in 1983 to institute a complex cost containment program with a revolutionary method of reimbursing hospitals for treating Medicare patients. The government agreed to pay hospitals in advance for each Medicare patient at a flat set rate for each of 468 diagnostic categories, called diagnosis-related groups (DRGs).

The goal of the program, aside from containing costs, was to give hospitals an incentive to be efficient and cost-conscious: money received from Medicare and not spent for care could be retained as a profit, but if costs exceeded the reimbursement for the treatment of a patient, the hospital would sustain a loss on that patient. The intent was to influence hospitals to stay within the limits set for each diagnostic category. When DRGs were put into practice, hospitals were still reimbursed for capital costs at cost. Although proposals to incorporate capital expenditures and the costs of medical education in the DRG payments were set forth by the Department of Health and Human Services in 1985, final arrangements on these issues were pending as this study was completed. Early critics of the DRG program suggested that it might lead to a decline in length of stay but to a rise in hospital admissions, but thus far the latter does not appear to have occurred.[42]

It is widely recognized that DRGs will require hospitals to be conscious of costs and to work actively with doctors to be sure that clinical treatment is administered with an eye to costs. The DRG program is shifting authority further away from physicians toward administrators, who are responsible for maintaining the fiscal solvency of hospitals. In most hospitals interdependence between administrators and physicians—shared authority—is the prevailing norm. And DRGs are bringing the federal government into the hospital decision-making process.

Hospitals that are accustomed to using extensive data collection and cost management decision making are likely to adjust more easily to the program. If hospitals perceive themselves as losing money under DRGs, they are expected to place limits on the intake of Medicare patients, shifting them to public hospitals, which have less discretion over admissions. This practice has not occurred, although hospital administrators and others in the industry, in conversations with the authors, have predicted that it will. DRGs are limiting the professional autonomy of doctors, insofar as their discretionary practices are being reviewed by local hospital administrators and by federal health care staff, who hold the purse strings.[43]

The first few years of DRG experience had mixed effects on hospitals. Some seemed to have higher margins than ever before, and some were sorely strapped. One effect for virtually all hospitals was that greater attention was paid to cost control and cost management.

With greater focus on cost control, many voluntary hospitals are confronting very explicitly the problem of how to finance care for the poor. During the past quarter-century, with cost reimbursement paramount, many hospitals had financed their charity and bad debt care by cost shifting; that is, they charged considerably higher rates to insured clients and used the extra money to finance charity care.[44] Although some disagreement exists over the scale of cost shifting, it was clearly a widespread practice that permitted hospitals to absorb bad debts, provide charitable care, and finance research and education indirectly.

Because the DRG program means the end of cost reimbursement for Medicare patients and other insurers have been driving harder bargains about reimbursement, cost shifting has been dramatically curtailed. Hospitals have found it increasingly difficult to find patients whose payers are willing to absorb higher rates than those charged to others. And without cost shifting there has been serious concern about how voluntary hospitals can continue to finance their charitable, research, and educational activities.

Some state regulatory programs have offered ways to fund uncompensated care in lieu of cost shifting. All-payer programs, under which all third parties are required to pay virtually the same amounts for care, were one possibility for spreading bad debt, charity, and other unreimbursable costs among all payers so that some do not carry a disproportionate share of the burden.[45] Other proposals and programs are discussed more fully in chapter 4. Some observers have taken the position that the costs of research, education, and charity in all hospitals should be explicitly recognized by society and paid for directly rather than indirectly by hospital users and their payers.

A major effect of cost-control regulation has been to stimulate in the voluntary hospital sector greater interest in being associated with other hospitals, through either networking arrangements or consolidation. An important goal has been to achieve economies of scale. Through cooperative arrangements, voluntary hospitals have been able to make less costly bulk purchases and to obtain better management expertise. Although free-standing voluntary hospitals have added experts to their staffs in a piecemeal fashion, they have found that more sophisticated staffing is available through cooperative efforts.[46]

40

A Transformation in the Hospital Environment. The American hospital industry has begun to experience a much more competitive and uncertain environment. As a result of vast technological changes, many diagnostic procedures can take place in the outpatient clinics of doctors rather than in hospitals. Various third-party payers have encouraged shifting service from the more expensive hospital site to less expensive alternatives. Whereas historically the doctor had provided hospitals with patients, certain medical specialists have now begun to compete with hospitals for patients.

By 1980 a widespread belief developed that the American hospital industry had considerable overcapacity as a result of the vast expansion in beds and hospitals during the past thirty years, the increasing complexity of state and federal regulation, the increased competition between doctors and hospitals, the expansion of organizations such as health maintenance organizations (HMOs) that ration hospital care, and the development of after-care centers designed to move patients quickly from acute-care hospitals. As early as 1973 hospital occupancy began to drop. Moreover, the days of hospital care per 1,000 population declined sharply during the late 1970s for every age group under sixty-five.

In 1984 the occupancy rate of voluntary hospitals in Chicago was approximately 50 percent. Dr. Sidney Lee, president of Michael Reese, the prestigious Chicago teaching hospital, commenting about overcapacity in the voluntary sector, said, "If Chicago lost forty voluntary hospitals tonight, no one would notice." This overcapacity, especially in large urban areas, made hospitals very competitive. In 1983 four-fifths of Chicago's voluntary hospitals experienced an operating loss, and 15 percent changed ownership. Bereft of their traditional philanthropic income and religious-ethnic ties, voluntary hospitals turned to more aggressive marketing tactics to attract patients.[47]

Some voluntary hospitals, especially small ones, found it increasingly hard to obtain capital for the replacement of depreciated equipment. The money available was constrained by the amounts recovered from third-party payers for equipment depreciation. Rising equipment costs and costly new technologies made it increasingly difficult for hospitals to rely on reimbursement to supply their equipment and technology needs.

Having substituted long-term borrowing for philanthropy as a means of raising capital, many small voluntary hospitals found by 1980 that depending on the bond market was problematic. Rising interest rates and declining prices of long-term bonds made many bond investors skeptical about investing in either long-term or intermediate bonds issued by voluntary hospitals. Investors became increasingly sensitive to the age and size of hospitals, their location, the

41

kinds of patients they served, the stability of their funding, the professional competence of administrators and chief financial officers, and the quality of medical staffs. Because it was difficult for many voluntary hospitals, especially small ones, to demonstrate that they ranked favorably on these indicators, their ability to acquire future capital through debt became clouded.[48]

As in any industry with threats of overcapacity, increasing and occasionally intense competition, shrinking financial resources, rapidly changing technology, and considerable uncertainty due to state and federal regulations affecting the stability of funding, efforts have been made to restructure the industry. This restructuring began to take place during the 1970s and 1980s—a subject discussed later in this chapter.

Public Hospitals

Environment, Origins, and Development

Almshouse origins. Public hospitals for acute care in the United States, as in Great Britain, emerged from circumstances quite different from those that gave rise to voluntary and proprietary hospitals. Initially, public authorities in the United States created social service institutions, such as prisons and hospitals for the mentally ill and the seriously contagious, mainly to protect society from those who were socially undesirable or dangerous.[49] Likewise, the very poor, those who seemed perennially dependent and unable to care for themselves, were granted a kind of miserable, minimal existence in almshouses provided by the state. The public purse might be opened, grudgingly, to care for people at a very low standard if private systems could not be found or if they posed some threat or embarrassment. But the provision was mean, and care received far less emphasis than custody. The earliest public hospitals emerged from this set of cultural expectations. No minority group was willing to provide care in the voluntary sector for certain "undeserving" groups, despite widespread agreement that something must be done. Under such conditions it was the state that was expected to act. Public authorities in nineteenth-century America, however, usually left to voluntary groups the provision of health services for the "deserving" poor.

The public institutions of the mid-nineteenth century customarily lacked separate facilities for those needing care for acute, chronic, or mental illness. Most were almshouses, which not only cared for the sick poor but also served as workhouses, jails, asylums, and homes for orphans. The public was generally indifferent about the quality of life in almshouses, which usually suffered a shortage of

42

funds, poor food, inadequate bedding and medicine, and untrained attendants.

In the long run city and county governments found it necessary to provide inmates with special facilities for medical care, including acute care, although they did so reluctantly. In crowded almshouses created for the "undeserving" poor, people fell ill, babies were born, and chronic diseases were commonplace. Under such circumstances, almshouses had to provide doctors and nursing, however unenthusiastically. The large institutions that were common because it was cheaper to batch-process the poor eventually had enough acute cases to merit a separate hospital. Thus public authorities that had not provided institutions for acute services began to supply them, but for the most part only to stigmatized classes. What they offered was a minimal-service facility for those who could not make their way to institutions provided by the voluntary or proprietary sectors.

Almshouses and the public hospitals that emerged from them were primarily a phenomenon of larger cities, not only in the East but also in western cities such as Denver, Los Angeles, and Seattle. But even after the public hospitals emerged as a separate institution, the stigma of the almshouse remained. Although many public hospitals eventually became predominantly acute-care facilities, their poorhouse origins were long remembered. Of course, a few cities developed public hospitals independent of almshouses that never had the stigma of the poorhouse. Two examples were the Cook County Hospital in Chicago and Boston City Hospital, both established in the 1860s.[50]

Public and voluntary hospitals, especially in larger cities, had a kind of symbiotic relationship. Once public authorities recognized an obligation to provide health care for the destitute, the trustees of voluntary hospitals felt even less obligation to treat such patients. They were less constrained from dumping patients if public facilities existed in the community. Hence the pressure to develop public hospitals was continuous, even after an extensive system of voluntary hospitals existed.

By the end of the First World War New York City had many voluntary hospitals, which had emerged in response to its heterogeneous population. The voluntary sector was either unable or unwilling to serve countless indigent citizens, however, although it was willing to accept public funds to serve a small proportion of them. As a result, New York City also developed by the 1920s an elaborate network of public hospitals for acute care. The system was quite varied, including both public hospitals famous for teaching and research and some that were little better than custodial.

In contrast, most large cities created one large municipal or county hospital. Some cities had separate public hospitals for blacks, such as the Kansas City Hospital, founded in 1930. Although conditions in public hospitals were generally far from ideal, their founding did reflect some governmental sense of responsibility for citizens who had no access to voluntary hospitals.[51]

Variations among large public hospitals before 1965. The extent to which large public hospitals have been mainly for the indigent has varied among regions. Public hospitals in larger, older metropolitan areas often originated in almshouses. Even after the almshouse was a thing of the past, public hospitals in the East continued to rely on public funding as their primary base of support. In western and somewhat newer parts of the country, many public hospitals did not emerge from the almshouse tradition. In the West, therefore, large public hospitals have not been stigmatized as outgrowths of the "poor law" tradition to the same degree as large eastern public hospitals. Serving the poor has long been common in the eastern public hospitals, whereas a larger proportion of public hospitals in the Far West have had more paying patients.[52]

We might ideally type public hospitals by the percentage of indigent patients. The larger the city, the more likely it would have multiple hospitals—several voluntary hospitals providing high-quality care for paying patients and one or more public hospitals providing care of lower quality primarily for the indigent.

Before the Second World War the means of financing large public hospitals varied from city to city. Throughout the country most large public hospitals collected fees from patients, but the expectation, especially in eastern cities, was that taxes would underwrite the bulk of the hospital budget. In some cities, large public hospitals attempted to limit their clientele to the indigent and admitted nonindigent patients only in emergencies. Sometimes municipal statutes limited care to the indigent, to prevent those who could pay from freeloading on the public facilities. In such circumstances private hospitals often refused charity cases with the argument that the special facilities for the poor should be used instead. A few public hospitals that insisted that those who could pay do so succeeded in elevating their status. Boston City Hospital did this from the beginning. By providing private rooms suitable for private patients, it enjoyed a better reputation than hospitals that catered predominantly to the indigent.[53]

Although the differences between large public and nonpublic hospitals have narrowed since the Second World War, their differences were earlier more pronounced. Obtaining their mandate from public authorities and more oriented toward the less fortunate than other kinds of hospitals, large public hospitals operated during the first several decades of the century under constraints different from those affecting other hospitals. Such hospitals, especially those designated for the indigent, had more mixing of acute-care patients with senile and chronic cases, less differentiation of short-term from long-term illness. More patients were alcoholics or social deviants or suffering from venereal disease—cases often rejected at voluntary hospitals. Voluntary hospitals of the late nineteenth and early twentieth centuries sometimes had clear policies against admission of some kinds of ailments and against charity patients, but large public hospitals rarely refused patients. They were recognized as institutions of last resort. Thus the state was responding to the needs of those for whom the voluntary and for-profit systems were unwilling to assume responsibility. Of course, public authorities—generally states rather than local governments—provided most of the institutions for the treatment of the tubercular and the insane.

Because they often depended on the public purse for funding and did not have patients of high socioeconomic status, large public hospitals often operated under very crippling financial constraints. The less the extent of service to poor people, the less the pressure on budgets. Most public hospitals were underfinanced and had chronically inadequate cash flows. Time and again before the Second World War, surveys demonstrated that expenditures per patient day were substantially higher in voluntary than in public hospitals. Of course, the inadequate funding affected the behavior of public hospitals. Many lagged behind voluntary hospitals in providing specialized services, in their standard of nursing, and in the extent to which they adhered to the prevailing standards of the day.[54]

The histories of large public hospitals are filled with stories of grotesquely crowded wards, of neglected patients waiting hours for care, of poor food and dirty linens. In 1873, for example, the Philadelphia Hospital had a capacity of 500 beds but had 1,000 patients, and the stench of patients poorly cared for was almost unbearable. As late as 1914 many patients at Charity Hospital in New Orleans were kept two to a bed.[55]

In an effort to improve the quality of American hospitals, the American College of Surgeons (ACS) instituted a program for evaluating hospitals during the First World War. The lack of ACS approval often stirred communities to address the inadequacies of their hospitals, and the periodic inspections did much to uplift the quality of public hospitals. Yet the history of the relationship between public hospitals and the ACS and other accrediting bodies has been one of recurring crises: the evaluating organization finding serious deficiencies, the hospital responding sufficiently to pass inspection, and later the hospital again falling below acceptable standards. In 1927, for example, the surveyors of the ACS reported that Cook County Hospital in Chicago was seriously deficient because of dirty wards, overcrowding, inadequate supplies, and substandard equipment. The hospital responded with reforms, but within a few years it was granted only provisional approval (in 1935, 1936, and 1937) and during 1938 lost its approval completely. In 1960 it was cited again, this time by the Joint Commission on Accreditation of Hospitals (JCAH), for having dirty, ill-kept, and overcrowded wards.[56]

Public hospitals in major cities were administered under a wide variety of governmental arrangements. Before the Second World War most were operated by cities and counties, not by special hospital or taxing districts. Some were jointly owned by a city and a county. Irrespective of the governing pattern, however, administrative arrangements were often complex, involving many levels of organization in all important decisions. In most cities such a fractionated system was cumbersome and inefficient. Rapid urban growth frequently led to administrative reorganization in municipal government, so that hospital governance responsibilities were passed from agency to agency.

Managed by local people, some public hospitals were especially subject to political influence and mismanagement, particularly where political machines existed. In such cities politicians occasionally viewed public hospitals as a source of employment for their relatives or cronies and in return expected loyal support in local elections from those employed in public hospitals. Purchasing for public hospitals was occasionally subject to manipulation and corruption. Kickbacks and rake-offs were not uncommon, and the selling of hospital goods illegally was not unknown. Moreover, political machines frequently interfered with the appointments of doctors to medical staffs.[57]

How political machines handled the hospital sector varied greatly, however. Mayor Curley, who dominated Boston politics before 1949 for some thirty-five years, gave the Boston City Hospital high priority. Believing that good medical care for the city was good politics, Curley did much to make certain that the hospital had high morale and a strong medical staff backed by affiliation with the Harvard and Tufts medical schools. At the same time Curley insisted that his henchmen and their families receive care without charge and treated nonprofessional positions as patronage positions.[58]

In Chicago the situation was quite different. Although machine politicians used Cook County Hospital to award contracts and to reward nonprofessional workers with patronage positions, the hospital was never given the high priority that Boston City Hospital received. Throughout the twentieth century Cook County Hospital has been plagued with poor morale and frequent problems with accrediting agencies. Shortly after the Second World War Boston City Hospital offered some of the finest medical care in the country, and its educational and research programs gained worldwide fame, while Cook County had annual expenditures of less than half those for Boston City Hospital, even though it had more patients. In contrast to Curley, Mayor Richard Daley of Chicago gave low priority to the quality of the public hospital. In 1955, when the Chicago police department suffered a serious lack of legitimacy, Daley searched the country for the leading police chief and made extensive reforms. But when Cook County Hospital came under fire from professional accrediting bodies, Daley paid very little attention.[59]

In major urban areas the appropriations for public hospitals frequently generated political controversy. Public hospitals for the indigent, with their dependence on tax dollars for almost the whole of their operating budgets, rarely had much influence in the political system. They were at the mercy of politicians, the bureaucracy, and the reformers, who were primarily interested in low costs and rarely gave high priority to distinction in performance. Moreover, members of the American medical profession have rarely expressed much concern for the well-being of large public hospitals. Most doctors have been preoccupied with their private practices, often struggling to find the time to keep up with technological changes, and have seemed to assume that those responsible for public hospitals must be capable of maintaining a high quality of care. At the same time most medical specialists have long known that this is not the case, because for many years a very high proportion of them were trained in large public hospitals.[60]

Obviously, large public hospitals should not be pictured as places of total neglect and incompetence. Clearly they were not. Some of the larger public hospitals, with their enormous intake of patients, resembled Boston City Hospital more than Cook County Hospital and were rich situations for teaching. They were able to attract excellent doctors who desired exposure to a vast array of cases. Although many public hospitals had no teaching affiliation, others were associated with medical schools, became important training grounds for doctors, and attracted extremely talented and creative staff. Even Cook County Hospital became one of the important centers in the country for training residents.[61]

Until the end of the nineteenth century almost all teaching hospitals in the United States were public hospitals. Among the more famous associations between public hospitals and medical schools were the arrangements between Los Angeles County Hospital and the medical school of the University of Southern California, between Baltimore City Hospital and Johns Hopkins Medical School, and between Boston City Hospital and the medical schools of Boston. Unfortunately, during most of the twentieth century Cook County Hospital has had very weak links with the medical schools of Chicago. The public hospitals affiliated with medical schools were unusual in the quality and quantity of their professional staff and often in their identity as tertiary-care facilities. They were protected and influenced by the medical schools rather than left primarily to the control of the politicians. As a result, they had a complex mission as well as a distinctive staff and funding pattern.[62]

Before the Second World War the large public hospitals that attracted the most attention were located in the nation's major cities. Cook County Hospital in Chicago at one time had 3,000 beds (plus bassinets) and was the largest acute-care hospital in the world. It was confined by statute to caring for the indigent and accepted paying patients only in emergencies. Yet size did not necessarily imply treating masses of patients inadequately. By 1940 the hospital had some notable achievements in teaching, even though previous and subsequent conditions were not always salubrious.[63] Philadelphia General, another large public hospital, provided care for the indigent with funding primarily from city taxes. Although private hospitals in Philadelphia also accepted needy patients, Philadelphia General was expected to bear the main load.

No system was nearly as complex as the New York City system. With more than twenty public general acute-care hospitals to administer, New York City has struggled throughout the twentieth century not only with problems of funding and quality but also with problems of control. There were really two separate issues: (1) what parts of the city government should be involved in setting policy for public hospitals; and (2) how the city government should hold the hospitals accountable for what occurred in them. Although these issues have been most intense and visible in New York, they have been persisting issues of public hospital governance in most large cities.[64]

Public hospitals outside metropolitan areas. Before the Second World War public hospitals outside metropolitan areas were usually rather different. In the first four decades of the century, if a small community did not have ethnic or religious minorities able to create a voluntary hospital, local governments often created a public hospital, financing it through the city's taxing power. In such communities city governments expected that patients' fees would fund most of the services but were prepared to pay for services for the indigent.

By the mid-1930s public hospitals had emerged in all regions of the country, accounting for 11 to 14 percent of the regions' general hospitals (see table 3). Until the end of the Second World War, moderate variation persisted among the regions of the country in the proportion of hospitals that were governmentally owned.[65]

During the 1930s most small communities either lacked or were unwilling to mobilize the resources to build a public hospital. Yet the demands on the public sector were considerable during the depression of the 1930s. Philanthropic giving, which had supplied approximately two-thirds of the capital for voluntary hospitals, virtually disappeared, at precisely the time that more and more patients were without the resources to pay for services. An increasing proportion of all patients turned to public hospitals and to the public sector for medical assistance. Faced with thousands of new patients, local public hospitals had little choice but to try to broaden their sense of mission. By bringing into sharp relief the fragility of voluntary and proprietary hospital systems and the lack of national health insurance, the depression heightened the national consciousness about the shortage of hospitals in many small communities, especially in states with low per capita incomes. After some years of debate about the inability of hundreds of local communities to finance hospitals and in response to pent-up wartime demand, the federal government responded in 1946 with the Hill-Burton program.[66]

When Congress held hearings on the program in 1946, there was widespread opposition to federal funding of proprietary hospitals. Partly because proprietary hospitals had been rather unstable in the past, closing down whenever the owner retired, died, or moved, there was widespread skepticism about their viability. More impor-

TABLE 3
HOSPITAL OWNERSHIP, BY REGION, 1935
(percent)

	Northeastern	Southern	Central	Western
Public hospitals	11	12	14	14
Voluntary hospitals	69	40	56	45
Proprietary hospitals	20	48	30	41

SOURCE: *Business Census of Hospitals, 1935*, p. 23.

TABLE 4

PUBLICLY OWNED HOSPITALS AS PERCENTAGE OF
NONFEDERAL GENERAL HOSPITALS, BY REGION, 1974

Region	Percent
Northeast	8
North-central	33
South	45
West	33

SOURCE: American Hospital Association, *1974 Statistical Profile of Public-General Hospitals* (Chicago: American Hospital Association, 1976).

tant, many Americans did not think it appropriate that hospitals should earn a profit from illness. Largely for these reasons, the Hill-Burton program denied federal funding for the construction of proprietary hospitals. As a result the number of public hospitals increased, and the number of proprietary hospitals decreased.

Although more Hill-Burton funding was used for voluntary than for public sector hospitals, more public hospitals were constructed. Many small towns and rural areas that had either no hospital or only a very small proprietary hospital received Hill-Burton funding for the construction of a small public hospital. The Hill-Burton program fundamentally transformed the American hospital industry. That program, more than any other factor, was responsible for the twofold increase in public hospitals, from 785 in 1946 to 1,704 in 1970. The distribution of public hospitals, which showed little variation among regions before the Second World War, had changed dramatically by the mid-1970s (see table 4). By 1975 approximately 31 percent of general hospitals were in the public sector.

States in which the greatest growth in hospitals occurred after the enactment of the Hill-Burton program usually had larger proportions of hospitals in the public sector, mostly located in small towns and rural areas. Thus by 1974 more than half the general hospitals in fifteen states were in the public sector. In states of the Rocky Mountain area and the Deep South, the public sector played a role in overcoming geographical barriers to hospital care. States in the Northeast already had a substantial supply of hospitals, mostly in the voluntary sector, and experienced relatively little expansion under the Hill-Burton program. The proportion of hospitals in the public sector in the Northeast was the lowest in the country.[67]

The Heterogeneity of the Public Hospital Sector. Largely because of the Hill-Burton program, the public hospital sector became increasingly heterogeneous. It is important to differentiate among four kinds of public general hospitals, which have different missions, structures, staffs, clientele, relations with other hospitals, financial conditions, sources of revenue, services, and educational programs. The four kinds are (1) large urban hospitals located in the nation's largest cities, (2) hospitals located in suburbs, standard metropolitan statistical areas (SMSAs), and cities other than the nation's 100 largest, (3) university-owned hospitals, and (4) hospitals in small towns and rural areas. Because these hospitals differ so substantially, it is desirable to highlight some of their recent characteristics.[68]

Large urban public hospitals. There are approximately ninety large public hospitals located in the 100 largest cities of the country. They face some of the most serious problems confronting hospitals in the United States.

These hospitals constitute 9 percent of the community hospitals in their cities, have an average of somewhat more than 500 beds, and in some cities provide one-third of all inpatient care and one-half of all outpatient care. Although they provide 5.5 percent of the nation's hospital care, they furnish 20.5 percent of its charity care. Moreover, they handle twice as many emergencies as the emergency departments of any other group of hospitals, and they have the highest percentage of total patient care attributable to outpatient services.[69] In contrast, large voluntary hospitals in these cities have enjoyed access to federal research funding, impressive philanthropic support, and highly qualified medical, research, and administrative personnel.[70]

Today, as in the past, many large public hospitals have attempted to serve the unprofitable patients who have been left over after private hospitals and physicians have claimed the more lucrative share of the medical market. True, voluntary hospitals have historically provided most of the services to the nation's poor. But the large urban public hospitals have served a disproportionately larger number of patients without third-party payers. Their share of Medicaid patients—both inpatients and outpatients—has been large; because Medicaid has paid less than full charges, this also posed problems for many of these hospitals. These hospitals have also served numerous low-income patients who have not been eligible for Medicaid and Medicare services. These have included (1) people who have earned too much in wages to qualify for public assistance but not enough to pay for medical care or medical insurance, (2) those who have had medical

51

insurance without adequate coverage for outpatient care, (3) the unemployed or the underemployed who, because of cutbacks in public assistance programs, have not qualified for welfare benefits, and (4) illegal aliens and nonresidents, who have not been eligible for public assistance.[71]

These hospitals have had higher proportions of poor patients than voluntary hospitals, irrespective of region or teaching status. The demands on them to serve nonpaying patients have increased in recent years as unemployment has increased and Medicaid rolls have been cut. But their financial resources have been very strained, since local governments have reduced their spending on medical services and third-party revenues have not expanded. Meantime, their financial problems have been aggravated as voluntary hospitals have increasingly been unwilling to treat uninsured patients or have dumped patients onto public hospitals through transfers. The result has often been acute financial stress. Since 1980 large public hospitals that provide 18 percent or more of their care to the poor have run chronic deficits and have been financially stressed.[72]

The demands on the large urban hospitals are even more complex. In the largest cities local governments have encouraged public hospitals to sponsor services or programs that the private sector has failed to provide. Thus the large public hospitals have provided a disproportionate share of burn centers, neonatal intensive care facilities, emergency services, and outpatient alcohol detoxification and treatment programs. These responsibilities have added to the possibility of financial stress.

In contrast with large public hospitals in sound financial condition, those that were financially stressed tended to be in communities with higher unemployment, a higher incidence of poverty, higher proportions of blacks and elderly people, less population growth, and poor city bond ratings.[73] Because of their social and regulatory environments, they have received less revenue from charge-paying commercial insurers (who often pay 30 percent more than costs) or from Blue Cross plans (which pay less than full charges but usually more than costs). Having too few commercially insured patients, some of these hospitals have been unable to generate sufficient financial surplus to cover the expenses of those receiving care without paying full costs.

It might appear that large public hospitals would have greater access to capital than private hospitals because of their ability to issue general obligation government bonds. In practice, however, those that have predominantly served poor patients have experienced considerable difficulty in raising capital in the nation's bond markets. Many have therefore found it difficult to carry out the renovations necessary to be in compliance with local codes.[74]

Most large public hospitals that are financially stressed have in recent years run deficits averaging 2 to 3 percent, and some have been in danger of having to close. Many have responded to their deficits by cutting back services, reducing quality, and giving up marginal activities—sometimes limiting care to charity patients. A few have closed or have been threatened with closure. Philadelphia General, one of the oldest public hospitals, closed in 1977, leaving that city without a public hospital. The Homer G. Phillips Hospital in St. Louis, which served the predominantly black North Side, closed in 1979. And New York City has seen continued public debate about the necessity of closing several public hospitals; four hospitals and parts of two others were closed between 1972 and 1977.[75]

Of course, the environment of large public hospitals in financial difficulty varies. Some have even greater problems because of state rate-setting regulations, as in New York during the 1970s. There Medicaid was tightly regulated, and hospitals were paid somewhat below their costs. Since physicians were paid approximately half the national average Medicaid fees, their participation in the state Medicaid plan was very low. In response large public hospitals used more salaried physicians and house officers rather than private physicians for care, causing their costs to be higher than those of hospitals without so many salaried doctors. Thus aspects of Medicaid rate setting contributed to the stressed financial condition of hospitals in New York and, to a lesser degree, in several other northeastern states.

During the 1970s New York's public hospitals were short of capital and, confined almost exclusively to indigent clients, in difficult financial circumstances. In response, the Health and Hospitals Corporation (an independent public corporation) undertook a tight management campaign, raised substantial capital, improved facilities, and made successful efforts to obtain payments for services to patients. The public hospitals also began to woo private paying clients and private practice doctors. Finally, with the all-payer plan in New York state covering all parties (including Medicare after 1983), financial arrangements were made by the state to cover uncompensated care. New York hospitals providing substantial charitable care were able to obtain reimbursement and thus to alleviate financial pressure. This relief was especially welcome to the public hospitals. How long this system will last is questionable, however.[76]

In some cities administrative problems have added further complications. The public hospital has been more complex and technical to manage than many other government agencies. Because many public hospitals have depended on public appropriations and have received third-party payments that were credited to local government accounts, they have never developed adequate internal systems of accounting, budgeting, billing, and collection. Some have depended on local governments for support services such as purchasing, maintenance, and data processing, but this has often hindered efficient, responsive operations. Moreover, the civil service requirements of some cities, intended to prevent inappropriate political influence, have had the unintended consequence of preventing some local hospitals from offering competitive salaries to managerial and technical staff.[77]

Because American society has long preferred the voluntary hospital and has tended to view large public hospitals as institutions for the indigent, it has consistently refused to give them adequate support. Bound by tradition, with "closed staff" who all too often have given higher priority to teaching than to good patient care, and often located in neighborhoods that lack political influence, large urban public hospitals have lacked the capacity to excel.[78]

In an effort to address their difficulties in acquiring high-quality medical staffs, an increasing number of hospitals have become more tightly integrated with university medical schools. Although affiliation of public hospitals with medical schools has a long tradition in the United States, the number of public hospitals affiliated with and subject to control by medical schools has dramatically increased in recent years.[79]

A complex set of motives have led to this process. From the viewpoint of the public hospitals, medical school affiliation has been a means of acquiring some of the high-quality staff found in private hospitals owned by or affiliated with private universities. The motives of the medical schools, however, have been much more complicated.

Most important, as medical specialties have become increasingly differentiated, medical schools have attempted to acquire a specialist in each specialty, so that the size of medical school teaching faculties has dramatically expanded. It has usually been necessary for the medical schools to increase the number of hospitals with which they have been affiliated. Because many hospitals have been separated by considerable distances, medical schools have often found it necessary to have duplicate services at each hospital.

Medical school departments have discovered, however, that one-person divisions are not academically viable. A single faculty member assigned to a subspecialty has usually found that he spends most of his time taking care of his clinical responsibilities and has no time for research. He often becomes disgruntled and tired; because he is not productive in research, he is not promoted. To cope with this problem, medical school faculties have increased each division by at least two people, so that they would have ample time to balance their responsibilities with clinical practice, teaching, and research. In some, the increases in the complexity of medical technology have led to a greater proliferation of medical subspecialties, which has led to more affiliation between medical schools and other hospitals in the same community.

This proliferation has substantially improved the quality of the medical staffs of the affiliated hospitals, many of which have been large urban public hospitals, but the affiliation has often posed problems for the clientele of the hospital. Not surprisingly, affiliation with strong medical and surgical subspecialties has frequently led to greater fragmentation, dehumanization, and discontinuity of services. Especially in complicated cases, good coordination in serving patients has generally been lacking, as patients have been shuttled from one hospital to another.

For basic services many of the urban poor have depended on the emergency rooms of large public hospitals, but medical school staffs have been unwilling to treat routine emergency room patients. As a result, despite the upgrading of the medical staffs of large urban hospitals, their emergency rooms and outpatient clinics are still overcrowded and inadequately staffed. A number of audits have found that a considerable difference persists in the quality of outpatient care received by low-income patients, who gravitate to the large urban hospitals, and that received by middle- and upper-income patients, who usually see physicians in their private offices.[80]

Public hospitals in other metropolitan areas. About 350 public hospitals are located in standard metropolitan statistical areas outside the nation's largest cities. A substantial majority of them are in affluent communities, and these are in the best financial condition of all public hospitals. Many have functioned as though they were in the private sector. In fact, some either have been managed by for-profit management companies or have been operated by voluntary corporations. Decision making in these hospitals, as in most voluntary hospitals, has been vested in the medical staff. Doctors in this kind of public hospital have usually not been salaried but have used the hospital as a place to send private patients.

These hospitals have derived a substantial portion of their revenues from commercial third-party payers and have had relatively few Medicaid and charity patients and very few bad debts. Some of them have had advantages over hospitals in both the for-profit and the voluntary sectors: they have had access to revenues from local tax systems and have been able to raise capital by issuing general-obliga-tion bonds through their government sponsors. Indeed, a few of these hospitals had been in the voluntary sector and became public sector hospitals simply to take advantage of the lower interest rates on tax-free government bonds.

Like the voluntary and for-profit hospitals in similar cities, these hospitals have for the most part been of medium size and have provided a full array of services. Thus they have required medical directors and chiefs of services. The medical staff has consisted pri-marily of physicians in private practice with attending privileges. Relatively few of the hospitals have been involved in training resi-dents or other health professionals.[81]

Public university-owned hospitals. There are forty-five public uni-versity hospitals, most located in the nation's largest cities. Because they have, with one exception, been owned by state governments, they have had a more secure financial base than most other large public hospitals in such cities. In addition to serving patients, they have had major missions in health science education and research. Partly as a result, they have often contained the most technologically complex and expensive equipment of any public hospitals. Many have been affiliated with other large public hospitals in the nation's major cities, and for that reason some effort is being made to coordi-nate specialization and expensive equipment with them. Because of their major teaching missions, they have kept abreast of the latest technological advances, often purchasing equipment and offering services less because of the needs of patients than because of their teaching relevance.

The medical staff in university hospitals, often composed of distinguished clinicians and researchers, has been very involved in hospital governance. Although professional administrators have been active in the management of such hospitals, they have usually de-ferred to the needs of medical divisions.

As the rate of growth in federal research funds has decreased, many public university hospitals have had to become more fiscally conservative in acquiring new equipment as well as in their teaching and research missions. Moreover, as unemployment has increased and Medicaid eligibility has been reduced, some of these hospitals have become more cautious in accepting charity patients.[82]

Public hospitals in small towns and rural areas. The most common kind of public hospital is in small towns and rural areas—constituting 71 percent of all public hospitals in 1982 but having only 4 percent of all public beds. Most of the hospitals have been small and have primarily provided general basic and ancillary services. Patients with
56

complex problems have usually been referred to larger hospitals for more specialized care. During the middle 1970s there were 664 public hospitals with fewer than fifty beds in small towns and rural areas. In many areas they were the only hospitals in the county, and for this reason their existence has historically been important in attracting physicians to small towns and rural areas. These hospitals have generally been staffed by physicians engaged in private practice. Most of them have not been affiliated with university medical schools and have not been involved in graduate medical training.

Unlike the large urban hospitals, whose financial problems resulted from the provision of a high volume of services to the poor, public hospitals in small towns and rural areas have provided much less service to the poor. Their financial problems have resulted largely from their small size and underuse. Their financial stress has tended to be less severe and less chronic. Only 20 percent of the smaller hospitals that ran deficits in 1980 ran them in three consecutive years, in contrast to 60 percent of the large urban public hospitals. The smallest hospitals have been more vulnerable to continued deficits, however, and must either improve their financial status or close. Approximately one-fourth of the financially stressed public hospitals in small towns and rural areas have been located in states with mandatory rate-setting programs, and some evidence suggests that such programs have contributed to financial problems.[83]

Summary. The public hospital sector has thus been very heterogeneous. Although most attention has focused on the large urban public hospitals that provide a disproportionate amount of care to the poor, most public hospitals are not located in the nation's largest cities, are relatively small, do not provide a disproportionate amount of care to the poor, and serve no teaching function. Yet the public hospital sector exists for reasons very different from those of hospitals in the private sector. Public hospitals have emerged in areas where the demands for collective goods are homogeneous and there has been considerable consensus about the role of a hospital. Where there are minorities or heterogeneously demanded public goods, voluntary hospitals have emerged. When minorities have wanted hospitals but have had insufficient capital to finance them, the public sector has provided a public hospital, but the source and amounts of funding for public hospitals have placed limits on their ability to fulfill their goals.

Proprietary Hospitals

Development from 1900 to 1965. The quintessential proprietary hospital in the early twentieth century was a result of two forces: lack of

57

local capital and physicians' preferences. Many small communities experienced difficulty in raising sufficient capital to fund a hospital. Even though hospitals founded at the beginning of the century were small and inexpensive by today's standards, capital was required to provide a building with some specialized facilities and to attract a nursing staff. Often not enough local capital could be mobilized collectively to meet even these modest requirements. Sometimes the community was too new or too small to include organizations that might take the lead in mobilizing the necessary capital. Especially in new and small communities, too few people had sufficient capital for a voluntary hospital to be a viable option. Even in some older communities, private capital was not available because of poverty. In such situations neither voluntary nor public hospitals emerged to meet local health needs.

In the late nineteenth century, most American cities had governments of limited scope. Urban governments supplied only minimal functions, such as police, fire, and public schools. Larger cities took some public responsibility for acute hospital services for the "deserving" poor, but this was generally not the response of small towns and villages. Before a small town would provide acute medical services, demand had to be widely expressed and shared, and it frequently was not. Occasionally, pesthouses were established to quarantine the poor who had contagious diseases. But the idea that a small town or village should provide a hospital at taxpayers' expense was generally not seriously considered.[84]

Although voluntary or public hospitals existed by 1910 in most cities with populations of 15,000 or more, many smaller communities could not fund such hospitals. If there were to be hospitals, they would have to be proprietary.

The preferences of doctors constituted the second force leading to the early and prolific development of proprietary hospitals. Doctors often preferred to group their more seriously ill patients in one location, to reduce the travel time needed to see them. A hospital built next to the doctor's office, even if it contained only a few beds, seemed to many physicians to permit more efficient practice as well as to provide a genuine social service. Hence, in advance of community demand for a hospital, doctors often believed that their communities and their professional practice required a hospital. Of course, proprietary hospitals were occasionally established in large cities, where some doctors had additional pragmatic motives for founding and administering them. They did not have hospital privileges at the existing hospitals and thus were in effect sending their patients to another doctor if they directed them to a hospital.[85]

58

Unlike European general practitioners, who have usually practiced outside hospitals, most American doctors have wanted to practice medicine in a hospital. If existing hospitals would not permit such arrangements, some doctors simply created their own. Indeed, the insistence of many American doctors in the twentieth century on having hospital privileges is an important reason why the United States eventually had more hospitals per capita than any other country in the world.

Often a lack of capital and physicians' preferences were combined. The local doctor most clearly perceived the need for a hospital and saw that if he did not create one, no one else would. By founding their own hospitals, doctors could be assured of keeping their patients who required hospitalization, not losing them to other physicians. If hospitals in large cities were inconveniently located or discriminated against some practitioners, doctors could expand their clientele and enhance their surgical skills by founding their own hospitals.[86]

Many lay people reasoned, Who better than a physician should run a hospital? If the hospital was located next to the doctor's office, as it often was, surely patients would receive more personal attention. Although doctors were usually the instigators and founders of proprietary hospitals, in a few instances groups of nurses, who wanted to provide a needed community facility, established hospitals.

Proprietary hospitals, as commonly organized in the 1890–1910 period, were very small, usually with a dozen or half a dozen beds. Often a house was turned into a hospital, with minor alterations to bathrooms and kitchen and the creation of an operating room. The sums necessary for converting a house to a hospital were modest enough that a small community might have five physicians and five hospitals (owned by those physicians).[87]

Regions varied considerably in the extent to which proprietary hospitals were founded. The intense poverty that prevented the emergence of hospitals sponsored by community groups was particularly notable in the southeastern United States. The same lack of community-sponsored hospitals in some mountain and Pacific coast states was due more to newness than to poverty. If no voluntary group began a hospital and at least a few patients with resources expressed a need for services, a for-profit hospital might be founded.

The proprietary hospital filled the needs of communities, patients, and physicians at low cost, developing in places in which there was not enough capital or perceived need for voluntary or government hospitals to originate. The proprietary form could be organized quickly and cheaply and thus fill a gap in the market flexibly and responsively. Its flexibility and responsiveness also permitted it to close if local support became too meager.[88]

The high turnover rates among proprietary hospitals suggest a certain lack of financial success. Indeed, there is very little evidence that proprietary hospitals were lucrative sources of income for their owners. No doubt some doctors hoped to benefit substantially from their investments, but there is no firm evidence that they did so.

Proprietary hospitals, as created in the late nineteenth and early twentieth centuries, were unpretentious enterprises, often carrying the names of their physician owners. Small as they were, they usually had no nursing schools or teaching affiliations. Supported primarily by patients' fees and without private endowments or tax subsidies, they had relatively short lives. The doctor who created the hospital might retire, die, or simply weary of the administrative load the hospital imposed. Arthur Hertzler, a renowned Kansas physician who created a proprietary hospital largely for his own convenience, found its administration an unending headache and regretted that he had to spend so much of his professional time on the mundane housekeeping details of hospital administration. Ultimately, after many years of hospital enlargement, he was delighted to sell his hospital to the Sisters of St. Joseph for $1.00. As Hertzler told it, he had not profited from the hospital—"not one thin dime." Patients' fees had all been used to maintain the hospital and to improve its facilities.[89]

Since proprietary hospitals were owned by doctors and often subsidized from the earnings of doctors, the key decisions in governing them were made by doctors. Most remained small enough to have no need for separate administrative staff; even if they did need such staff, the supremacy of the medical staff remained unquestioned.

During the 1930s and 1940s federal hospital surveys found what individual accounts had recorded earlier: proprietary hospitals were less enduring, with fewer years of operating experience, than public and voluntary hospitals.[90] Like for-profit firms in general, proprietary hospitals did not find it difficult or cumbersome to go out of business. They simply closed. There were no trustees to consult, no public authorities who had to approve. In metropolitan areas doctors who chose to move to the suburbs following their middle-class patients could divest themselves of their hospitals without much effort. Because proprietary hospitals tended to be small, there was not much pressure in most communities to keep them open to fulfill community responsibilities. When such pressures emerged, the hospitals were frequently transformed into public or voluntary hospitals.[91]

The evidence regarding the quality of these hospitals is very limited. Because they were very small, they were generally not subject to inspection by the American College of Surgeons. When the American Medical Association in 1928 found 458 hospitals unworthy of inclusion in their registered list of medical institutions, 67 percent were proprietary hospitals. Clearly, the American Medical Association viewed proprietary hospitals as of substantially inferior quality to those in the voluntary or public sectors.[92]

The conditions leading to the emergence of proprietary hospitals did not wholly disappear as the twentieth century advanced. As communities grew and prospered, however, voluntary groups frequently became sufficiently organized to raise capital for hospitals, so that proprietary hospitals became less common. If voluntary hospitals did not emerge, the demand for a hospital led to the creation of more public hospitals. During the first third of the twentieth century, more and more doctors were able to obtain privileges at existing hospitals, so that having one's own hospital became less necessary to keep paying clients.[93]

Proprietary hospitals could not truly fill the needs of the community. Their reluctance to accept many charity patients perpetuated the need for facilities for the indigent.[94] And their limited capacity to raise capital meant that they could not respond to rapidly developing need in fast-growing communities or to the ever-changing medical technology.

The proprietary hospitals were especially hard pressed by the depression of the 1930s. As thousands of Americans who had relied on proprietary hospitals for care were unable to pay their medical bills, hundreds of proprietary hospitals closed. Some were taken over by the voluntary and public sectors, but most simply disappeared.

The decline in proprietary hospitals was not continuous everywhere. After the Second World War new constellations of population developed rapidly in California, Texas, and Florida. As in earlier decades, new communities often lacked the social, economic, and political infrastructure necessary to create voluntary or public hospitals. Usually, however, there was some demand—even though small—for a hospital to provide acute care. The newness of these areas meant that for-profit hospitals were quick to develop, confident that there would be enough paying patients to keep them open and to protect investors. Indeed, during the twenty years after the Second World War, proprietary hospitals grew far more rapidly in areas where the population increased substantially and hardly at all where the population was relatively stable. Steinwald and Neuhauser concluded that proprietary hospitals proliferated where the demand for hospitals outstripped the capacity of the nonprofit system to accommodate it.[95]

As in former times, however, proprietary hospitals in new areas sometimes lost their favored positions as voluntary or public community hospitals emerged. Other proprietary hospitals located in suburbs of expanding metropolitan areas were able to thrive and expand. Groups of doctors usually furnished the capital for the hospitals, for by the late 1940s hospitals had become far too expensive for a single physician to capitalize.[96]

Before 1965 proprietary hospitals functioned at the margin of the medical delivery system, although in some regions they were important providers. In the South, for instance, by 1950 a sizable percentage of hospitals were proprietary, in contrast to the very small percentages in the New England and middle Atlantic states. In 1968 almost two-thirds of proprietary hospitals were located in five states—Texas, California, Louisiana, Tennessee, and New York. Ten states, five in New England, had no such hospitals. By the mid-1960s only 14.9 percent of all nonfederal short-term general hospitals were proprietary, in contrast to approximately 56 percent in 1909 and 36 percent in 1935. Furthermore, only 6 percent of general hospital beds were in the proprietary sector in 1965 in contrast to 13 percent in 1935.[97]

The Changing Environment of Proprietary Hospitals. Beginning in 1965, however, the federal government, through the Medicare and Medicaid programs, revitalized the proprietary hospital industry. During the 1970s the share of all general hospital beds in for-profit hospitals began to increase rapidly, after falling for several decades. By 1983 there were more beds in the proprietary sector than ever before.

Although some observers have seen the strength of the proprietary sector as due to the fact that for-profit organizations always enjoy more vitality than nonprofit ones—particularly governmental institutions—the proprietary hospital sector would probably have continued its long-term decline without the infusion of federal money. First, Medicare and Medicaid agreed to reimburse proprietary hospitals—like public and voluntary hospitals—for interest on debt as well as for costs of depreciating plant and capital equipment. Second, Medicare reimbursement guaranteed for-profit hospitals a reasonable return on equity as part of the hospital cost base. Because public and voluntary hospitals did not receive a return on equity, Medicare gave proprietary hospitals certain distinct advantages. The return on net equity has varied, but it has occasionally been as high as 20 percent. Before

1982 return on equity was set at 1.5 times the rate earned on investments of the Medicare Hospital Insurance Trust Fund. Since 1982 it has been equal to the rate earned by the Medicare trust fund.[98]

Whereas voluntary hospitals enjoy such incentives as relief from corporate taxation, ability to receive tax-deductible gifts, and no obligation to distribute profits to shareholders, for-profit hospitals have received other advantages. Various federal and state taxes have been allowable costs under the Medicare program, reducing the advantages of tax-exempt nonprofit hospitals over for-profit hospitals. And while voluntary nonprofit hospitals have been able to float tax-exempt bonds and thus to acquire higher bond ratings and pay lower rates of interest, tax-exempt financing has also been available under limited circumstances to investor-owned hospitals under the so-called small issue exemption. Investor-owned hospitals have also raised capital by issuing stock—a strategy that has been unavailable to public and voluntary hospitals. Finally, lower taxes and milder regulatory climates in southern states have been incentives for proprietary hospitals.

Federal funding for proprietary hospitals through the Medicare and Medicaid programs constituted a marked change from the circumstances when Hill-Burton was enacted some two decades earlier. As Kenneth Arrow and others have pointed out, the idea of profit making by hospitals has historically aroused suspicion on the part of patients and referring physicians. Both have preferred nonprofit institutions, in either the voluntary or the public sector.[99] In recent years, however, American proprietary hospitals have slowly acquired enhanced legitimacy for a variety of reasons.

Changes in the funding pattern. With the passage of Medicare and Medicaid legislation, proprietary hospitals could be substantially reimbursed for treating patients to whom they had not previously directed much service. With an enlarged pool of paying patients available thanks to federal entitlement programs, proprietary hospitals enlarged and improved their services to attract patients. Since the Medicare reimbursement formula made capital expansion financially possible, they were able to become much more like voluntary hospitals. They competed for charge-paying patients and enlarged their medical staffs. Moreover, once Medicare came into effect, voluntary hospitals no longer had such large charity burdens and thus became more like proprietary hospitals in their reliance on patients whose care was paid for by third parties. As voluntary and proprietary hospitals became more alike, the proprietary sector gained a bit more legitimacy.

More general recognition that all hospitals seek profits. Although it has long been understood that proprietary hospitals were operated for profit, in the past two decades it has become increasingly clear that voluntary and public hospitals have similar motives. Their desire is to acquire reserves, a form of profit, which have become an important source of capital expansion in the past decade.[100] The recognition that hospitals of all ownership types attempt to earn profits has made the proprietary hospital seem less unusual and hence more legitimate.

The extensive regulation of all hospitals. Once for-profit hospitals became closely regulated by local, state, and federal regulatory agencies as well as by professional accrediting bodies, their legitimacy was also considerably advanced. Greater regulation occurred in part because of their participation in the Medicare program. Although criteria for opening and operating hospitals continued to vary from state to state, national standards have become matters of relatively routine application in proprietary hospitals.

Efforts to placate staff physicians from the community. No longer were proprietary hospitals the small appendage of a single physician's practice, with perhaps fewer than a dozen beds. For many years their size has been increasing, as they have shifted more and more from being owned by a single person to corporate status. As they have acquired corporate status and grown, many of their features have converged with those of voluntary hospitals.

Increasingly, both kinds of hospitals have been managed by professional administrators who attempt to please their staff physicians. In all three sectors medical staffs have played important roles in governing hospitals. Physicians have largely determined the quality of hospital care and have decided whether patients are admitted. The hospital administrator may have primary responsibility for billing and collecting, purchasing, laundry, and material management, but the administrator cannot compel physicians to admit patients. By maintaining an efficient operation and by catering to the needs of a medical staff, however, the administrator can attract physicians and patients. Once proprietary hospitals became larger and independent of the owner-physician and had to generate the respect of a diversified medical community, their respectability increased, even though their owners were investors uninvolved in the practice of medicine. A proprietary hospital cannot expect to incur the displeasure of the medical community and remain profitable. As proprietary hospitals made serious efforts to respond to physicians' preferences, their legitimacy in medical circles was significantly enhanced.[101]

Despite the enhanced legitimacy of proprietary hospitals, controversy still clouds their existence. On one side Arnold Relman, editor of the prestigious *New England Journal of Medicine*, echoed the sentiments of many in a 1983 editorial suggesting that large corporate for-profit hospitals have been less cost effective than their nonprofit counterparts and have inadequately served the public interest.[102] Certainly proprietary hospitals have a history of serving relatively few charity patients and engaging in little medical research or teaching.

Others contend that proprietary hospitals have engaged in "cream skimming"—that is, they have generally attempted to serve patients with substantial third-party coverage and to avoid services with high unit costs that are little used.[103] These allegations are difficult to document; there is anecdotal documentation but little research demonstrating that cream skimming is a systematic practice of proprietary hospitals. Nevertheless, proprietary chains have much greater flexibility than nonprofit hospitals in where they may be located, and for this reason they have tended to be located where more prosperous and relatively well-to-do patients reside. In recent years, however, as they have acquired better management, they have often offered some special services that are not much used. This they have done as a result of more aggressive marketing and careful scheduling.[104] Moreover, they have become more active in medical education and research, taking advantage of the Medicare pass-through system for reimbursement.

In the meantime the legitimacy of proprietary hospitals has been further enhanced by the burgeoning literature arguing that they are more efficient than nonprofit hospitals. A number of economists, for example, more for theoretical than for empirical reasons, believe that the proprietary sector is more efficient because it has the appropriate incentives to be responsive to rapidly changing market forces in the health area. Moreover, proprietary hospitals are alleged to be more efficient because they can achieve economies of scale through effective centralized planning, management, and marketing.[105] As the discussion in the next chapter demonstrates, however, some evidence suggests that proprietary hospitals are no more efficient than voluntary hospitals.

Multi-institutional Arrangements

The For-Profit Sector. Since the early 1960s the proprietary hospital sector in the United States has been fundamentally restructured. At that time most proprietary hospitals were free-standing institutions, owned either by individuals or by small, privately held partnerships or corporations. Most of the owners were physicians. By the middle

1970s, however, the vast majority of these hospitals had been sold to large corporations whose stock was traded on various stock exchanges. Medicare's reimbursement system encouraged mergers by making them financially rewarding and thus contributed to the dramatic consolidation.

Many of the free-standing proprietary hospitals needed new capital to meet the standards for participation in the Medicare program. Moreover, many owners of free-standing institutions did not want to cope with the complex government regulations required by the Medicare program. As a result, many physicians in the South and West decided to sell their interests to for-profit hospital chains rather than continue to finance and operate the hospitals independently.[106] Of course, the proprietary sector was not the first in which considerable consolidation of the hospital sector existed, for many Catholic and other religious hospitals had long been integrated into systems, but the dramatic and rapid consolidation of the proprietary sector attracted much attention.

By 1982 approximately 80 percent of all proprietary hospital beds were part of proprietary chains—defined as organizations owning and operating three or more hospitals. Indeed, proprietary chains were the fastest growing phenomenon in the American hospital industry in the late 1970s. The number of proprietary hospitals in chains grew more than 100 percent between 1973 and 1982 (from 317 to 668) while the number of beds increased almost 150 percent (from 36,976 to 89,171). Chains grew primarily by purchasing other proprietary hospitals rather than by acquiring voluntary or public hospitals. The growth of chains was generally greatest in regions where proprietary hospitals already had a large share of the beds, where there were rapid increases in population, per capital income, and insurance coverage, and where hospital rate regulation was weakly developed;[107] that is, in the Sunbelt. Frostbelt areas had an ample supply or oversupply of voluntary and public sector hospitals and had historically had few proprietary hospitals. By and large proprietary chains were attempting to acquire hospitals that were often poorly managed and to improve their efficiency.

Although there were about three dozen proprietary hospital chains in 1980, four corporations had acquired at least two-thirds of all investor-owned short-term hospital beds in the United States. They were Hospital Corporation of America (HCA), Humana, American Medical International (AMI), and National Medical Enterprises (NME). The companies varied somewhat in their structures and operating strategies.

HCA was very much involved not only in owning but also in

managing hospitals in all three sectors. It was distinguished by decentralized management, whereby the local hospital had considerable autonomy but was expected to meet specified performance criteria. In 1985 HCA owned or managed 422 health care facilities, had revenues of $4.1 billion and profits that had grown for a number of years by more than 20 percent, and managed hospitals in more than half a dozen foreign countries. Beginning in 1983, however, the federal government imposed a new system—based on diagnosis-related groups (DRGs)—of reimbursing hospitals for Medicare patients, which apparently limited the earning potential of proprietary hospitals. As a result HCA's earnings from hospitals became rather flat in 1985 after many years of impressive growth, prompting industry analysts to speculate that HCA and some other large chains might reduce their hospital business.[108]

In contrast, Humana's hospitals were subject to tight centralized control, with especially strict controls over revenues and expenses. Humana was primarily involved in the ownership of hospitals. Because of its centralized structure, it could quickly respond to changes in the economic climate and new opportunities. Humana, like most for-profit chains, raised capital for acquiring hospitals mostly by borrowing rather than by issuing stock or by spending from revenues.

To recruit the doctors it wanted, Humana occasionally put up office buildings near its hospitals and offered doctors subsidized rents. It recruited doctors from across the country and occasionally guaranteed them their first-year salaries. As part of its centralized data, it kept a record of every doctor's monthly admissions and the revenues produced. Unlike HCA, Humana responded quickly to the DRG program by diversifying into other medical industries, particularly into medical insurance.

In 1980 NME was the most diversified of the large proprietary chains. It owned as well as managed hospitals, and it was the only major hospital management company that owned nursing homes. Moreover, it was diversified into construction and purchasing services as well as into medical products and equipment distribution. AMI also sold services to other hospitals: laboratory and pharmaceutical services, respiratory and physical therapy, CT scanners, and alcohol treatment centers. AMI and NME were based in California, Humana and HCA oriented more to the South.[109]

As the regulatory and reimbursement environment has become more complex, the traditional free-standing hospital in all three ownership patterns has faced new strains. The increasingly complex environment, the inefficiency of many small, free-standing hospitals, and the financial incentives of the federal government have provided an opportunity for restructuring much of the American hospital industry. As a result of their size, large proprietary hospital chains have increasingly been able to develop specialized skills to match the highly differentiated hospital environment. They acquired specialists in third-party reimbursement, legal problems related to hospital regulation, labor relations, recruitment of physicians, quality assurance, purchasing of equipment and services, financial management and capital markets, construction and building management, and systems development. Having acquired these skills, they have been in a strategic position to market them to hospitals in all three sectors too small to afford highly specialized management.[110]

Subject to centralized management decisions, doctors practicing in investor-owned hospitals have, at least theoretically, been likely to exercise less influence in local hospitals. Although the findings are mixed on this point, staff physicians apparently consider themselves very much involved in all critical decisions concerning the quality of care, and thus far doctors recruited by investor-owned hospitals appear to be treated very deferentially.[111]

Historically, hospitals were able to cope with their local environment through personal contacts and subjective criteria. Internally, local hospitals were managed through an unsystematic and paternalistic system of rewards and punishments. In recent years, however, a folksy and local orientation has given way to a highly complex and differentiated reimbursement system for determining payment. Hospitals have found it increasingly necessary to develop sophisticated measures of performance and to resort to market criteria to perform well. The traditional and personalistic systems of rewards and punishments have yielded to more systematic ones with universalistic criteria. Facing mounting regulatory and competitive pressures, hospitals have found it necessary to develop highly complicated and bureaucratic skills to cope with an increasingly uncertain environment. As they have become more complex internally, they have had to acquire more sophisticated managerial skills to coordinate the various parts. Because proprietary hospitals have greater flexibility in altering goals, structure, and strategies, it should not be surprising that they have been the most successful in developing economies of scale, in coping with external markets, in acquiring highly specialized managerial skills, and in moving quickly into areas with lucrative markets.[112]

The large investor-owned hospital companies have attempted to be uninvolved in areas, services, and clients that fail to produce profits. Nevertheless, because large proprietary companies have good access to capital markets and the ability to recruit physicians, some

68

communities with investor-owned hospitals have acquired more specialized and higher quality services than they would otherwise have had.

Nonprofit Hospitals: The Public and Voluntary Sectors. The hospital industry has employed a variety of strategies to respond to its changing environment. First, some hospitals have merged with one another into a single organization, mimicking the chains prevalent in the proprietary hospital sector. Second, some hospitals wishing to retain a bit more autonomy have combined with others through federations or have become part of holding companies. Third, several hundred hospitals in all three sectors, wishing to retain even greater autonomy, have entered into contracts under which they have remained separate legal entities but have received the specialized services of a management company. Fourth, the most common multi-institutional arrangement has consisted of hospitals sharing services with other hospitals. This arrangement has involved the least structural change and has permitted the free-standing hospital to retain the most autonomy.[113]

The extent to which hospitals in the three sectors have been able to use these four models varies. Both the constraints of the sector and local circumstances may make some options more viable than others. Hospitals in the public sector have the least capacity to engage in mergers or to become part of holding companies or federations. A voluntary hospital in Florida may merge with a group of voluntary hospitals in Texas or California. Most Catholic hospitals have some form of collective association, as do Seventh-Day Adventist hospitals, most Lutheran hospitals, and voluntary hospitals making up various regional organizations: the Fairview Community Hospitals, the Greenville Hospital System, and the like.[114] But New York City's public hospitals cannot merge with the public hospitals in Los Angeles and remain in the public sector.

The large urban public hospitals, embedded in complex political systems, lack the flexibility to adapt to changing environmental conditions. Not only are they constrained by complex political forces, but they are also hampered by their age and size. As Forrester and others have demonstrated, the larger and older an organization, the more impervious it becomes to environmental changes and the more it resists structural and policy changes.[115] Enjoying fewer options than voluntary and proprietary hospitals to cope with a rapidly changing health industry, public hospitals have resorted most frequently to loose affiliations with other hospitals, shared services, and management contracts.

Shared services are an important means by which hospitals have sought to control costs without eliminating services. By 1980 approximately 80 percent of hospitals shared services, with an average of 6.2 services shared. The sharing of services is obviously more common among hospitals in urban areas than among those in small towns and rural areas. Because so many public hospitals are in small towns and rural areas, sharing services is more common among voluntary than among public hospitals.[116] The services shared most frequently include blood banks, data processing and billing services, and the professional staffs in laboratories. But the most common sharing has been in purchasing of medical and surgical supplies.

Most free-standing hospitals very much want to preserve their autonomy and have entered into arrangements with other hospitals somewhat reluctantly. Over time, however, as they have entered into alliances with neighboring hospitals for shared services, the distrust of trustees and medical staffs has decreased. Modest sharing of services has slowly increased the willingness of community hospitals to become integrated into larger systems, usually first by increasing the services and facilities shared with other organizations and later by resorting to more systematic and tightly integrated systems.

Increasingly, trustees and medical staffs of small free-standing hospitals have recognized that their management base is too thin to cope with all the complexities of the American hospital industry. Hospital management companies have argued that they can provide the management and administrative expertise unavailable in the free-standing hospital, which finds itself almost daily in some crisis, and that they can improve the finances of the hospital through more aggressive billing of third-party payers.

Because the DRG program subjects the hospital to considerable pressure for high-quality data on costs and utilization, it has especially emphasized the need for efficient hospital management. Since contract management agreements exist for short periods and pose little threat to the autonomy and control of board members or to the identity and ownership of local hospitals, they have become an effective way of reconciling the demands for collective expertise with the demand for continued independence and autonomy.

Hospitals having one or more of the following characteristics have been the primary users of contract management: deficit operation; chronic low occupancy; small town, rural, or very large urban location; small size (fewer than 200 beds); location in an area having trouble attracting skilled administrators; aging facilities, with outdated structures that have badly deteriorated; or location in a newer community that does not have well-established groups to support a hospital.[117]

TABLE 5

CHARACTERISTICS OF HOSPITALS UNDER CONTRACT MANAGEMENT,
1980

	All Hospitals		Small Hospitals		Large Hospitals	
	No.	%	No.	%	No.	%
Type of hospital						
Public (nonfederal)	173	40.1	129	49.0	44	26.2
Religious	39	9.0	17	6.5	22	13.1
Other nonprofit	196	45.5	102	38.8	94	56.0
Investor owned	23	5.3	15	5.7	8	4.8
Total	431	100.0	263	100.0	168	100.0
Urban-rural						
Rural	285	66.1	207	78.7	78	46.4
Urban	146	33.9	56	21.3	90	53.6
Total	431	100.0	263	100.0	168	100.0

NOTE: Small hospitals are those with fewer than 100 beds; all others are in the large category.
SOURCE: Compiled from Jeffrey A. Alexander and Bonnie L. Lewis, "Hospital Contract Management: A Descriptive Profile," *Health Services Research*, vol. 29 (October 1984).

Small hospitals in both the voluntary and the public sectors have especially needed the skills of external management. They have frequently had occupancy rates of 50 to 60 percent, have been under pressure to close their obstetric and pediatric units (or have already done so), and have had considerable difficulty in mastering all the complex code regulations and reimbursement schemes (see table 5). Although 300 beds is considered the optimal size for maximum economies of scale, more than half the hospitals in the United States in 1980 had fewer than 100 beds, and hospitals with fewer than 200 beds constituted somewhat more than two-thirds of the total. These hospitals in the public and voluntary sectors were having great difficulty in adjusting to their rapidly changing medical environment and were in need of contract management.[118]

For a while contract management was dominated by aggressive for-profit hospital chain companies, which had entered the management business for several reasons. First, contract management was an effective means of developing greater depth and specialization in managerial skills. Second, it extended their knowledge into new geographical markets and gave them intimate knowledge about hospitals with which they might wish to merge. Finally, it was lucrative, with high returns on existing investment.

In more recent years voluntary nonprofit hospitals—particularly those that have developed large systems and strong management of their own—have also moved into the contract management business. Indeed, some of the largest systems in the voluntary sector have behaved very much like investor-owned chains in the management business.[119]

Thus far little evaluation has taken place of hospitals under contract management, involving very few cases and extending over a very limited period. Preliminary results suggest, however, that governing boards of such hospitals have experienced high satisfaction. Trustees of smaller hospitals, in particular, believe that many complex problems have been more skillfully handled through contract management.[120]

Considerable concern has been expressed, however, that management contracting may have driven away needy clients who could not afford to pay for care, eliminated costly services that were not fully reimbursed by third-party payers or patients, increased the costs of services, and emphasized high-return services, such as surgery and laboratory tests, at the expense of those that yield low returns. Unfortunately, little information is available about contract management to respond adequately to these concerns. Shonick and Roemer found that contract management did not reduce hospital operating costs during the era before DRGs. Moreover, there is no evidence that it has led to a deterioration in inpatient services, although there is very modest evidence that it has led to some improvement in the quality of care.[121]

The free-standing American hospital increasingly participates in multi-institutional arrangements or networks that extend across sectors and organizational types. A centrally managed, for-profit hospital might have a management contract to operate a voluntary hospital that shared services with another voluntary hospital and had obtained capital through a decentralized affiliated system. Both the affiliated system and the for-profit company might have grown vertically by adding other kinds of hospitals and health facilities. Moreover, the for-profit company might have merged with profit-making firms to provide supplies to hospitals or entered into real estate development. An interesting network, or hybrid, is Voluntary Hospitals of America, a for-profit company whose shareholders include over seventy large nonprofit hospitals.[122]

Many other mixtures can be imagined, involving cross-sectoral links, vertical and horizontal growth, and both short- and long-term arrangements. The hospital sector is beginning to behave like other sectors of the economy, becoming an industry trying to use the language and tools of management without losing the legitimacy derived from its historical sense of mission and obligation to persons who are ill.

The implications and dynamics of multihospital arrangements are not well understood since most of the changes have taken place in less than twenty years. It is easy to exaggerate the extent to which the traditional hospital sector has been modified. Some dynamics, however, seem relatively clear:

• Consolidation and system development have occurred rapidly in all three sectors, fueled by societal pressures to contain costs and by the possibilities that management information systems provide for detailed, rapid financial analysis. Among voluntary and for-profit hospitals, multi-institutional arrangements have enhanced concentration. Concentration is, of course, already well advanced in the proprietary sector and is moving apace in the voluntary sector. The public sector is the least concentrated and is likely to remain decentralized.[123]

• In this era of consolidation and rationalization, small hospitals, especially those in urban areas, are in considerable peril of closure. Hospitals in small towns and rural areas may be better able to survive if they assume clearly understood roles as satellite hospitals.[124]

• There may be less sensitivity to community needs and conditions if hospitals, traditionally constrained by local boards of trustees or local officials, continue to affiliate or merge with systems having their headquarters elsewhere.[125]

• Because multi-institutional arrangements vary in the extent to which they are centralized, their effect on hospital governance is mixed. Size of system, geographic dispersion, cultural expectations, and other factors shape the extent to which systems become centralized and thus the extent to which nonresident technocrats assume authority over decisions having clinical implications, which historically were left to the discretion of physicians.

• Increased consolidation has permitted somewhat easier access to capital markets for participating hospitals and at lower costs than for free-standing hospitals.[126]

• Since the costs of acquiring hospitals are very high, it is unlikely that new chains of investor-owned hospitals will develop. The financial requirements are simply too great for another HCA or Humana to emerge. There is evidence that the managers of these organizations believe that they already have excessive investments in American hospitals.[127]

• Regulation and federal pressure, which have already wrought so much change in hospitals, are continuing to increase, generating even further pressures for consolidation, particularly in the voluntary non-profit sector, although much of the earlier consolidation took place in the for-profit sector.[128]

• The restructuring of the voluntary and for-profit hospital systems is continuing to increase faster than its consequences can be understood. Starkweather has estimated that mergers take from fifteen to twenty-five years to achieve their predicted efficiencies. Because the cost savings attributed to mergers and management contracts are poorly understood, the pace of structural change appears to be greater than evaluations and cost-benefit analysis would warrant.[129]

• There are indications that vertical integration is becoming an increasingly important strategy among voluntary and for-profit hospitals in large metropolitan areas, as the squeeze on profit margins requires them to look outside acute care for additional revenues. For some large hospitals, especially in the voluntary sector, strategies of forward and backward links have been selected to enhance cash flow. Some hospitals have attempted to operate satellite clinics and to create health maintenance organizations to ensure a flow of clients. Some have established free-standing emergency care facilities. Forward links include the provision of nursing homes, home health care services, and even hospices. Other expansion has taken the form of office buildings for doctors, supported living facilities for infirm or handicapped persons, and diagnostic or special-function technical facilities. Many hospitals in all three sectors have developed "fitness" programs as the hospital environment becomes increasingly competitive. In short, hospitals have developed many strategies to find new markets and customers. Besides vertical integration, hospitals have resorted to joint ventures, informal networks, and interlocking directorships to reduce uncertainty and to improve coordination with other organizations. Because public hospitals have had much less flexibility than for-profit or voluntary hospitals, they have been much less involved in pursuing strategies with other kinds of organizations.[130]

• Business management and cost control measures combined with more price competition have had a substantial effect on the amount of charitable care that public and voluntary hospitals provide. Aware of the costs of charitable care and increasingly unable to shift costs to meet them, the hospitals have been subject to financial pressures to reduce certain kinds of services.[131] Because of cost pressures by large purchasers of care, hospitals are likely to have even less ability to finance charitable care in the future. Historically, voluntary hospitals used much of their philanthropic revenue to finance charitable care; but as costs have risen, they have used their philanthropic dollars for capital expenditures. Hence, a conscious trade-off has been made between charitable and capital expenditures. As this has occurred, the belief that hospital care is a community responsibility has declined. American society increasingly views hospitalization as a commodity.

• Reviews of the literature indicate that hospitals in systems may have made more efficient use of personnel than independent hospitals but did not perform more efficiently. System hospitals did not cost less than independent hospitals and, indeed, appear to have cost more for patient care. System hospitals exhibited much the same quality as independent hospitals. There is hard-fought disagreement on these points, some of which are discussed below.[132]

• The diffusion of highly skilled management throughout all three sectors has meant that management style is becoming more comparable among hospitals of comparable size. Whether similar management practices will cause performance among hospitals in the three sectors to converge is still problematic—a problem discussed in the chapter that follows.

Notes

1. Jeff Charles Goldsmith, *Can Hospitals Survive?* (Homewood, Ill.: Dow Jones–Irwin, 1981), p. 107.

2. See the articles by Louis Block in *Modern Hospital*, 1956 and 1959.

3. See the following very useful studies: Charles E. Rosenberg, "Inward Vision and Outward Glance: The Shaping of the American Hospital, 1880–1914," in David J. Rothman and Stanton Wheeler, eds., *Social History and Social Policy* (New York: Academic Press, 1981), pp. 19–55, and the longer version in *Bulletin of the History of Medicine*, vol. 53 (1979), pp. 346–91; Charles E. Rosenberg, "The Hospital in America: A Century's Perspective," in *Medicine and Society: Contemporary Medical Problems in Historical Perspective* (Philadelphia: American Philosophical Society, 1971); Paul Starr, *The Social Transformation of American Medicine* (New York: Basic Books, 1982); Morris J. Vogel, *The Invention of the Modern Hospital: Boston, 1870–1930* (Chicago: University of Chicago Press, 1980); David Rosner, *A Once Charitable Enterprise* (Cambridge: Cambridge University Press, 1982); Leonard Eaton, *New England Hospitals, 1790–1837* (Ann Arbor: University of Michigan Press, 1957), p. 26; and David Rosner, "Heterogeneity and Uniformity: Historical Perspectives on the Voluntary Hospital," in Bruce Vladeck, ed., *Future Mission of Voluntary Health Care Institutions* (New York: United Hospital Fund, 1987). For additional sources on the founding of hospitals, see note 6 in Rosenberg, "Inward Vision and Outward Glance."

4. Morris J. Vogel, "The Transformation of the American Hospital, 1850–1920," in Susan Reverby and David Rosner, eds., *Health Care in America* (Philadelphia: Temple University Press, 1979), pp. 105–16; Rosenberg, "Inward Vision and Outward Glance"; Eaton, *New England Hospitals*, p. 237; Eric

Larrabee, *The Benevolent and Necessary Institution: The New York Hospital, 1771–1971* (Garden City, N.Y.: Doubleday, 1971), pp. 107, 202; Starr, *Social Transformation*; Rosemary Stevens, "'A Poor Sort of Memory': Voluntary Hospitals and Government before the Depression," *Milbank Memorial Fund Quarterly*, vol. 60 (1982), pp. 551–84; and Rosner, *A Once Charitable Enterprise*, p. 18.

5. Rosenberg, "Inward Vision and Outward Glance."

6. J. M. Toner, "Statistics of Regular Medical Associations and Hospitals of the United States," *Transactions of the American Medical Association*, vol. 24 (1873), pp. 314–33.

7. Jon Michael Kingsdale, "The Growth of Hospitals: An Economic History in Baltimore" (Ph.D. dissertation, University of Michigan, 1981), vols. 1 and 2; Rosner, *A Once Charitable Enterprise*; Starr, *Social Transformation;* and Rosenberg, "Inner Vision and Outward Glance."

8. Rosemary Stevens, "Voluntary and Governmental Activity," *Health Matrix*, vol. 1 (Spring 1985), p. 27.

9. Rosner, *A Once Charitable Enterprise;* and Vogel, *Invention of the Modern Hospital*.

10. Larrabee, *Benevolent and Necessary Institution*, p. 202; Joan E. Lynaugh, "The Community Hospitals of Kansas City, Missouri, 1870–1915" (Ph.D. dissertation, University of Kansas, 1982), pp. 29–30; Charles Perrow, "Authority, Goals, and Prestige in a General Hospital" (Ph.D. dissertation, University of California, Berkeley, 1960); and Rosner, *A Once Charitable Enterprise*, p. 17.

11. Joseph Hirsh and Beka Doherty, *The Mount Sinai Hospital of New York* (New York: Random House, 1952); and Starr, *Social Transformation*.

12. Michael M. Davis and C. Rufus Rorem, *The Crisis in Hospital Finance* (Chicago: University of Chicago Press, 1932), chap. 2.

13. "The Chronological Development of the Catholic Hospital of the United States and Canada," *Hospital Progress*, vol. 4 (April 1940), pp. 122–33.

14. James A. Hamilton, *Patterns of Hospital Ownership and Control* (Minneapolis: University of Minnesota Press, 1961), p. 90; Warren L. Johns and Richard H. Utt, eds., *The Vision Bold* (Washington, D.C.: Review and Herald Publishing Association, 1977); Dorothy Levenson, *Montefiori: The Hospital as Social Instrument, 1884–1984* (New York: Farrar, Straus and Giroux, 1984); and Perrow, "Authority, Goals, and Prestige."

15. Emily Friedman, "Private Black Hospitals," *Hospitals*, vol. 55 (July 1981), pp. 65–68; and Samuel Rodgers, "Kansas City General Hospital No. 2," *Journal of the National Medical Association*, vol. 54 (September 1962), pp. 527–35.

16. Stevens, "A Poor Sort of Memory," p. 557; and Vogel, *Invention of the Modern Hospital*.

17. Harvey S. Perloff, Edgar S. Dunn, Jr., Eric E. Lampard, and Richard F. Muth, *Regions, Resources, and Economic Growth* (Lincoln: University of Nebraska Press, 1960), pt. 3.

18. Kingsdale, "Growth of Hospitals"; and Vogel, *Invention of the Modern Hospital*, and "Transformation of the American Hospital."

19. Starr, *Social Transformation*.

20. Stevens, "Voluntary and Governmental Activity," p. 28.

21. See Vogel, "Transformation of the American Hospital," and *Invention*

of the Modern Hospital; Rosner, *A Once Charitable Enterprise;* and David Rosner, "Business at the Bedside: Health Care in Brooklyn, 1890–1915," in Reverby and Rosner, *Health Care in America,* pp. 117–31.

22. Rosner, *A Once Charitable Enterprise,* chap. 3.

23. U.S. Department of Commerce, *Benevolent Institutions, 1904* (Washington, D.C., 1905).

24. Stevens, "A Poor Sort of Memory," pp. 551–84; S. S. Goldwater, "The Appropriation of Public Funds for the Partial Support of Voluntary Hospitals in the United States and Canada," *Transactions of the American Hospital Association,* vol. 11 (1909), pp. 242–94; Kingsdale, "Growth of Hospitals"; Starr, *Social Transformation,* p. 173; and Robert Dripps, "The Policy of State Aid to Private Charities," *Proceedings of the National Conference on Charities and Corrections,* May 12–19, 1915, pp. 458–73.

25. Margaret L. Plumley, "Payments from Tax Funds to Voluntary Hospitals for Out-Patient Service," *Hospitals,* vol. 14 (January 1940), pp. 99–102; and Michael Davis, "The Indigent Patient and the Voluntary Hospital," *Hospitals,* vol. 13 (July 1939), pp. 32–35.

26. Lucy Freeman, *Hospital in Action* (New York: Rand McNally, 1956).

27. Herman M. Somers and Anne R. Somers, *Doctors, Patients, and Health Insurance* (Washington, D.C.: Brookings Institution, 1961); Walter J. McNerney and Study Staff, *Hospital and Medical Economics,* 2 vols. (Chicago: Hospital Research and Educational Trust, 1962); Odin W. Anderson, *The Uneasy Equilibrium: Private and Public Financing of Health Services in the United States, 1875–1965* (New Haven, Conn.: College and University Press, 1968); and U.S. Public Health Service, *Health Statistics from the U.S. National Health Survey,* series B, no. 30, tables 25–27, pp. 38–40.

28. Lewis E. Weeks and Howard J. Berman, *Shapers of American Health Care Policy: An Oral History* (Ann Arbor, Mich.: Health Administration Press, 1985), pp. 145–48; Odin W. Anderson, *Blue Cross since 1929: Accountability and the Public Trust* (Cambridge, Mass.: Ballinger, 1975); Sylvia Law et al., *Blue Cross: What Went Wrong?* (New Haven, Conn.: Yale University Press, 1974), chap. 1; Robert D. Eilers, *Regulation of Blue Cross and Blue Shield Plans* (Homewood, Ill.: Richard D. Irwin, 1968), pp. 83–84; Somers and Somers, *Doctors, Patients,* chap. 15; and Theodore R. Marmor, Mark Schlesinger, and Richard W. Smithey, "A New Look at Nonprofits: Health Care Policy in a Competitive Age," *Yale Journal of Regulation,* vol. 3 (Spring 1986), pp. 323–25.

29. Law et al., *Blue Cross,* pp. 7–20; Weeks and Berman, *Shapers,* pp. 137–44; Anderson, *Blue Cross since 1929,* p. 98; Eilers, *Regulation of Blue Cross,* pp. 3–31; and conversation of authors with Robert M. Cunningham, Jr., consultant to Blue Cross Association/Blue Shield Association, December 3, 1985.

30. Anderson, *Blue Cross since 1929;* and Marmor et al., "New Look at Nonprofits," pp. 327–28.

31. U.S. Department of Health, Education and Welfare, *Facts about the Hill-Burton Program,* July 1, 1947–June 30, 1971; *Hill-Burton Progress Report, 1970–1971;* James F. Blumstein, "Court Action, Agency Reaction: The Hill-Burton Act as a Case Study," *Iowa Law Review,* vol. 69 (July 1984), pp. 1227–61, and "Providing Hospital Care to Indigent Patients: Hill-Burton, A Case Study and Paradigm," in Frank A. Sloan, James F. Blumstein, and James M. Perrin, eds.,

Uncompensated Hospital Care: Defining Rights and Assigning Responsibilities (Baltimore: Johns Hopkins University Press, 1985).

32. Judith R. Lave and Lester B. Lave, *The Hospital Construction Act: An Evaluation of the Hill-Burton Program, 1948–1973* (Washington, D.C.: American Enterprise Institute, 1974); Dan Feshbach, "What's inside the Black Box: A Case Study of Allocative Politics in the Hill-Burton Program," *International Journal of Health Services*, vol. 9 (1979), pp. 313–39; and Institute of Medicine, *Controlling the Supply of Hospital Beds* (Washington, D.C.: National Academy of Sciences, 1976).

33. Carolyne K. Davis, "Effects of Medicare, Medicaid on Community Hospitals," *Hospital Finance Management*, vol. 36 (July 1982), pp. 34–38.

34. Starr, *Social Transformation*, pp. 375, 387–88; and Martin S. Feldstein, *Hospital Costs and Health Insurance* (Cambridge, Mass.: Harvard University Press, 1981).

35. Paul Lawrence and Davis Dyer, *Renewing American Industry* (New York: Free Press, 1983), pp. 86–116.

36. For a discussion of these functions of voluntary hospitals, see Richard W. Foster, "The Nonprofit Hospital: Evolution and Future Prospects" (unpublished paper, University of Colorado at Denver, September 1983); Starr, *Social Transformation;* and Anderson, *The Uneasy Equilibrium.*

37. Judith Feder and Bruce Spitz, "The Politics of Hospital Payment," *Journal of Health Politics, Policy, and Law,* vol. 4 (Fall 1979), pp. 435–63.

38. Frank A. Sloan, "Rate Regulation as a Strategy for Hospital Cost Control: Evidence from the Last Decade," *Health and Society,* vol. 61 (1983), pp. 195–222; and Gail H. Klapper and Rebecca L. Harrington, "Viewpoint: The Rise and Fall of Cost Containment in Colorado," *Health Care Management Review,* vol. 6 (Spring 1981), pp. 79–83.

39. Thomas W. Bice, "Health Planning and Regulation Effects on Hospital Costs," *Annual Review of Public Health,* vol. 1 (1980), pp. 137–61; D. S. Salkever and T. W. Bice, "The Impact of Certificate-of-Need Controls on Hospital Investment," *Health and Society,* vol. 54 (1976), pp. 185–212; D. S. Salkever and T. W. Bice, *Hospital Certificate-of-Need Controls: Impact on Investment, Costs, and Use* (Washington, D.C.: American Enterprise Institute, 1979); and Louise B. Russell, *Technology in Hospitals: Medical Advances and Their Diffusion* (Washington, D.C.: Brookings Institution, 1978).

40. Office of Planning, Evaluation, and Legislation, *Professional Standards Review Organizations: Program Evaluation–Executive Summary* (Washington, D.C.: Health Services Administration, U.S. Department of Health, Education and Welfare, 1978); A. Dobson, J. G. Greer, R. H. Carlson, F. A. Davis, L. E. Kucker, B. J. Steinhardt, T. P. Ferry, and G. S. Adler, "PSROs: Their Current Status and Their Impact to Date," *Inquiry,* vol. 15 (1978), pp. 113–28.

41. Nancy L. Worthington and Paula A. Piro, "The Effects of Hospital Rate-setting Programs on Volumes of Hospital Services: A Preliminary Analysis," *Health Care Financing Review,* vol. 4 (December 1982), pp. 47–65; "Rate Regulation," *Topics in Health Care Financing,* vol. 6 (Fall 1979), pp. 1–140; Michael A. Morrisey, Frank A. Sloan, and Samuel A. Mitchell, "State Rate Setting: An Analysis of Some Unresolved Issues," *Health Affairs,* vol. 2 (Summer 1983), pp. 36–47; Glenn Melnick, John R. C. Wheeler, and Paul J. Feld-

stein, "Effects of Rate Regulation on Selected Components of Hospital Expenses," *Inquiry,* vol. 18 (1981), pp. 240–46; Craig Coelen and Daniel Sullivan, "An Analysis of the Effects of Prospective Reimbursement Programs on Hospital Expenditures," *Health Care Financing Review,* vol. 2 (1981), pp. 1–40; Paul Joskow, *Controlling Hospital Costs: The Role of Government Regulation* (Cambridge, Mass.: MIT Press, 1981); Frank A. Sloan, "Regulation and the Rising Cost of Hospital Care," *Review of Economics and Statistics,* vol. 63 (1981), pp. 479–87; and Sloan, "Rate Regulation as a Strategy."

42. Andrew B. Dunham and James A. Morone, *The Politics of Innovation* (Princeton, N.J.: Health Research and Educational Trust of New Jersey, 1983); Richard F. Averill and Michael J. Kalison, "Prospective Payment by DRG," *Hospital Finance Management,* vol. 35 (February 1983), pp. 12–14, 18, 20, 22; John S. Cook, Marvin Rushkoff, and Richard J. Henley, "Hospital Prospective Rate Setting Principles and Their Application," *Hospital Finance Management,* vol. 35 (December 1983), pp. 60–68; Gilbert S. Omenn and Douglas A. Conrad, "Sounding Board: Implications of DRGs for Clinicians," *New England Journal of Medicine,* vol. 311 (November 15, 1984), pp. 1314–17; John Wennberg, Kim McPherson, and Philip Caper, "Will Payment Based on Diagnosis-related Groups Control Hospital Costs?" *New England Journal of Medicine,* vol. 311 (August 2, 1984), pp. 295–300; *New York Times,* March 12, 1984; and *New York Times,* August 26, 1984.

43. Stephen M. Shortell, "Physician Involvement in Hospital Decision Making," in Bradford Gray, ed., *The New Health Care for Profit* (Washington, D.C.: National Academy Press, 1983), pp. 73–101; *New York Times,* May 30, 1982; Paul Ellwood, "When MDs Meet DRGs," *Hospitals,* vol. 57 (December 16, 1983), pp. 62–66; and James W. Bjorkman, "Politicizing Medicine and Medicalizing Politics: Physician Power in the United States" (Paper prepared for European Consortium for Political Research, Barcelona, Spain, March 25–30, 1985). For further discussion of the recent changes in the control of hospitals, see Victor R. Fuchs, *The Health Economy* (Cambridge, Mass.: Harvard University Press, 1986), chap. 15.

44. Charge patients are those who pay a share of the hospital's total expenses for operation (including bad debt and charity as well as debt costs, depreciation, and medical costs). Cost patients pay less, with third-party payers refusing to share in charitable, bad debt, research, and some other kinds of expenses.

45. See Douglas Conrad et al., "All-Payer Rate Regulation: An Analysis of Hospital Response," in Marion Ein Lewin, ed., *The Health Policy Agenda: Some Critical Questions* (Washington, D.C.: American Enterprise Institute, 1985), pp. 65–84; Jack Hadley and Judith Feder, "Troubled Hospitals: Poor Patients or Management," *Business and Health,* vol. 1 (September 1984), pp. 15–19; Jack Hadley and Judith Feder, "Hospitals' Financial Status and Care to the Poor in 1980" (Washington, D.C., Urban Institute, October 1983), Executive Summary; Judith Feder, Jack Hadley, and Ross Mullner, "Falling through the Cracks: Poverty, Insurance Coverage, and Hospital Care for the Poor, 1980 and 1982," *Health and Society,* vol. 62 (1984), pp. 544–66; Jack A. Meyer, *Passing the Health Care Buck: Who Pays the Hidden Cost?* (Washington, D.C.: American Enterprise Institute, 1983); and Paul B. Ginsburg and Frank A. Sloan, "Hospi-

tal Cost Shifting," *New England Journal of Medicine,* vol. 310 (April 5, 1984), pp. 893–94.

46. Frank A. Sloan, "Property Rights in the Hospital Industry," in H. E. Frech III, ed., *Health Care in America: Political Economy of Hospitals and Health Insurance* (San Francisco: Pacific Research Institute for Public Policy, forthcoming); Robert Derzon, Lawrence S. Lewin, and J. Michael Watt, "Not-for-Profit Chains Share in Multihospital System Boom," *Hospitals,* vol. 55 (May 16, 1981), pp. 65–71; Joseph S. Coyne, "'Networking' Enhances Viability of Not-for-Profit Multihospital Systems," *Hospitals,* vol. 55 (August 16, 1981), pp. 123–30; and Jeffrey Alexander and W. Richard Scott, "The Impact of Regulation on the Administrative Structure of Hospitals," *Hospital and Health Services Administration,* vol. 29 (May/June 1984), pp. 71–85.

47. American Hospital Association, *Hospital Statistics, 1984 Edition* (Chicago: American Hospital Association, 1984), p. xvii; Jeff Goldsmith, "Death of a Paradigm," *Health Affairs,* vol. 3 (Fall 1984), pp. 5–19; interview with Dr. Sidney Lee, president of Michael Reese Hospital, Chicago, Illinois, March 23, 1984; and interview with Howard Cook, director of Chicago Hospital Council, March 24, 1984.

48. Reed Stigen, "Methods for Financing Capital Projects," *Hospital Finance Management,* vol. 35 (April 1983), pp. 11–16; and Ross Mullner, Dale Matthews, Joseph D. Kubal, and Steven Andes, "Debt Financing: An Alternative for Hospital Construction Funding," *Hospital Finance Management,* vol. 35 (April 1983), pp. 18–24. See also Geoffrey B. Shields, ed., *Debt Financing and Capital Formation in Health Care Institutions* (Rockville, Md.: Aspen Systems, 1983).

49. Brian Abel-Smith, *Value for Money in Health Services* (London: Heinemann Educational Books, 1976), chap. 7; and J. Rogers Hollingsworth and Ellen Jane Hollingsworth, "Differences between Voluntary and Public Organizations: The Behavior of Hospitals in England and Wales," *Journal of Health Politics, Policy, and Law,* vol. 10 (Summer 1985), pp. 371–97.

50. Harry F. Dowling, *City Hospitals* (Cambridge, Mass.: Harvard University Press, 1982); Toba Schwaber Kerson, "Almshouse to Municipal Hospital: The Baltimore Experience," *Bulletin of the History of Medicine,* vol. 55 (1981), pp. 203–20; Kingsdale, "Growth of Hospitals"; *Transactions of the American Hospital Association,* vol. 11 (1909), pp. 242–94; David J. Rothman, *The Discovery of the Asylum* (Boston: Little, Brown, 1971); Mary Risley, *The House of Healing: The Story of the Hospital* (Garden City, N.Y.: Doubleday, 1961); and Judith W. Leavitt, *The Healthiest City: Milwaukee and the Politics of Health Reform* (Princeton, N.J.: Princeton University Press, 1982).

51. Haven Emerson, *The Hospital Survey for New York* (New York: United Hospital Fund, 1937), vols. 1, 2, 3; and Rodgers, "Kansas City General Hospital."

52. Ivan Belknap and John G. Steinle, *The Community and Its Hospitals: A Comparative Analysis* (Syracuse, N.Y.: Syracuse University Press, 1963), p. 35.

53. Elizabeth J. Davis, "History, Development, and Organization: Cook County Hospital," *Chicago Hospital Council Bulletin,* vol. 8 (September 1945), pp. 7–14, 20; and Dowling, *City Hospitals,* pp. 32–83, 151.

54. Kingsdale, "Growth of Hospitals"; S. S. Goldwater, "The United States

Hospital Field," *National Hospital Record*, vol. 9 (April 1906), p. 11; *Hospital Management*, vol. 23 (July 1927), p. 51; and Dowling, *City Hospitals*, pp. 149–50.

55. Charles K. Mills, "The Philadelphia Almshouse and the Philadelphia Hospital from 1854 to 1908," in John W. Croskey, ed., *History of Blockley: A History of the Philadelphia General Hospital from Its Inception, 1731–1928* (Philadelphia: W. A. Davis, 1929); Albert E. Fossier, "The Charity Hospital of Louisiana," *New Orleans Medical and Surgical Journal*, vol. 76 (September 1923), pp. 136–38; and Dowling, *City Hospitals*, p. 78.

56 Rosemary Stevens, *American Medicine and the Public Interest* (New Haven, Conn.: Yale University Press, 1971); Dowling, *City Hospitals*, pp. 93–94, 107–8, 146–48, 176; Illinois Legislative Investigating Commission, *Cook County Health and Hospitals Governing Commission* (Chicago: State Government of Illinois, 1980); and Milton I. Roemer and Jay W. Friedman, *Doctors in Hospitals: Medical Staff Organization and Hospital Performance* (Baltimore: Johns Hopkins University Press, 1971).

57. Ray E. Brown, "The Public Hospital," *Hospitals*, vol. 44 (July 1, 1970), pp. 40–44; Lynaugh, "Community Hospitals"; Amos Warner, *American Charities* (New York: Arno, 1971), pp. 370–80; Vogel, *Invention of the Modern Hospital*; and Thomas N. Bonner, *Medicine in Chicago* (New York: Stratford Press, 1957).

58. John J. Dowling, "Plans and Progress of the Boston City Hospital," *New England Journal of Medicine*, vol. 198 (May 24, 1928), pp. 723–24.

59. Illinois Legislative Investigating Commission, *Cook County Commission*; and Dowling, *City Hospitals*, pp. 92–98, 146.

60. Milton I. Roemer and Jorge A. Mera, "'Patient-Dumping' and Other Voluntary Agency Contributions to Public Agency Problems," *Medical Care*, vol. 11 (January–February 1973), p. 36; Stevens, *American Medicine and the Public Interest*; and Dowling, *City Hospitals*, pp. 135–36.

61. Lewis Thomas, *The Youngest Science* (New York: Viking Press, 1983).

62. Brown, "The Public Hospital"; Helen E. Martin, *The History of the Los Angeles County Hospital, 1873–1968, and the Los Angeles County–University of Southern California Medical Center, 1969–1978* (Los Angeles: University of Southern California Press, 1979), p. 164; Kerson, "Almshouse to Hospital"; and Kenneth M. Ludmerer, *Learning to Heal: The Development of American Medical Education* (New York: Basic Books, 1985).

63. Davis, "Cook County Hospital"; and Illinois Legislative Investigating Commission, *Cook County Commission*.

64. Nathan Sinai and Alden Mills, *A Survey of the Medical Facilities of the City of Philadelphia, 1929* (Chicago: University of Chicago Press, 1931); Charles E. Rosenberg, "From Almshouse to Hospital: The Shaping of Philadelphia General Hospital," *Health and Society*, vol. 60 (1982), pp. 108–54; David Rosner, "Gaining Control: Reform, Reimbursement, and Politics in New York's Community Hospitals, 1890–1915," *American Journal of Public Health*, vol. 70 (1980), pp. 533–42; Emerson, *Hospital Survey*; Samuel Wolfe, Fred Goldman, and Hila Richardson, "The Fiscal Crisis of New York City: The Conflict in Allocation of Resources to the Public and Private Health Sectors," *Consumer Health Perspectives*, vol. 6 (1980), pp. 1–6; Robb K. Burlage, *New York City's Municipal Hospitals: A Policy Review* (Washington, D.C.: Institute for Policy Studies,

1967); and Robert R. Alford, *Health Care Politics: Ideological and Interest Group Barriers to Reform* (Chicago: University of Chicago Press, 1975).

65. McNerney and Study Staff, *Hospital and Medical Economics*, vol. 1, p. 9. See the papers and references in Ronald L. Numbers and Judith Walzer Leavitt, eds., *Wisconsin Medicine: Historical Perspectives* (Madison: University of Wisconsin Press, 1981); and Joseph W. Mountin, Elliott H. Pennell, and Evelyn Flook, "Hospital Facilities in the United States: Selected Characteristics of Hospital Facilities in 1936," *Public Health Bulletin*, no. 243 (Washington, D.C., 1938), p. 11.

66. Davis and Rorem, *Crisis in Hospital Finance;* and Risley, *The House of Healing*, p. 221.

67. See notes 31 and 32.

68. For further discussion of contemporary public general hospitals, consult Hospital Research and Educational Trust, *Report of the Commission on Public-General Hospitals* (Chicago: Hospital Research and Educational Trust, 1978); and E. Richard Brown, "Public Hospitals on the Brink: Their Problems and Their Options," *Journal of Health Politics, Policy, and Law*, vol. 7 (Winter 1983), pp. 927–44.

69. American Hospital Association, *1974 Statistical Profile of Public-General Hospitals* (Chicago: American Hospital Association, 1976); and Margaret B. Sulvetta, "Public Hospital Provision of Care to the Poor and Financial Status" (Washington, D.C., Urban Institute, 1985).

70. Wolfe, Goldman, and Richardson, "Fiscal Crisis," p. 2.

71. Brown, "Public Hospitals on the Brink"; and Hospital Research and Educational Trust, *Report on Public-General Hospitals*, p. 17.

72. Sulvetta, "Public Hospital Care"; Judith Feder, Jack Hadley, and Ross Mullner, "Poor People and Poor Hospitals: Implications for Public Policy," *Journal of Health Politics, Policy, and Law*, vol. 9 (Summer 1984), pp. 237–50; Feder, Hadley, and Mullner, "Falling through the Cracks"; Hadley and Feder, "Hospitals' Financial Status"; Roemer and Mera, "Patient-Dumping"; Brown, "Public Hospitals on the Brink"; Gordon Schiff, "Letter to the Editor," *New England Journal of Medicine*, vol. 312 (June 6, 1985), p. 1522.

73. Hadley and Feder, "Hospitals' Financial Status in 1980," p. 61.

74. Hospital Research and Educational Trust, *Report on Public-General Hospitals*, pp. 31–32.

75. Brown, "Public Hospitals on the Brink," p. 927; David B. Starkweather, *Hospital Mergers in the Making* (Ann Arbor, Mich.: Health Administration Press, 1981), p. 7; and Dowling, *City Hospitals*, p. 185.

76. Hadley and Feder, "Hospitals' Financial Status in 1980," pp. 65–70. For a discussion of efforts to confront some of these problems in New York, see Jack A. Meyer, "Financing Uncompensated Care with All-Payer Regulation," in Sloan, Blumstein, and Perrin, *Uncompensated Hospital Care;* interview with Vice President Pamela S. Brier of the New York City Health and Hospitals Corporation, April 11, 1986; Judith Graham, "City System's Changes Help It to Win Respect," *Modern Healthcare*, vol. 15 (May 24, 1985), pp. 50–58; and New York City Health and Hospitals Corporation, *Annual Report*, 1984.

77. Hospital Research and Educational Trust, *Report on Public-General Hos-*

pitals, pp. 26–28. Jack Hadley and Judith Feder, however, take the position that financial stress cannot be explained by differences in management practices.

78. Stephen M. Weiner and Dorothy Pugh, "Requisites for a Sound Fiscal Policy for the Large Urban Public-General Hospital," *Readings on Public-General Hospitals* (Chicago: Hospital Research and Educational Trust, 1978), pp. 359–60.

79. Ludmerer, *Learning to Heal*.

80. Robert G. Petersdorf, "The Evolution of Departments of Medicine," *New England Journal of Medicine*, vol. 303 (August 28, 1980), pp. 489–96; Eli Ginsberg, *Urban Health Services* (New York: Columbia University Press, 1971); Burlage, *New York City's Hospitals;* and Robert A. Derzon, "The Politics of Municipal Hospitals," in Douglas Cater and P. R. Lee, eds., *The Politics of Health* (New York: Medcom Press, 1972).

81. Hospital Research and Educational Trust, *Report on Public-General Hospitals*.

82. Ibid.

83. Ibid.; Hadley and Feder, "Hospitals' Financial Status," Executive Summary; and Sulvetta, "Public Hospital Care."

84. J. Rogers Hollingsworth and Ellen Jane Hollingsworth, *Dimensions in Urban History* (Madison: University of Wisconsin Press, 1979).

85. Starr, *Social Transformation*, pp. 146–69; and Carson W. Bays, "Patterns of Hospital Growth: The Case of Profit Hospitals," *Medical Care*, vol. 21 (September 1983), pp. 850–57.

86. Lynaugh, "Community Hospitals," p. 37; and Vogel, *Invention of the Modern Hospital*, pp. 102–4.

87. Arthur Hertzler, *The Horse and Buggy Doctor* (Lincoln: University of Nebraska Press, 1938).

88. Bruce Steinwald and Duncan Neuhauser, "The Role of the Proprietary Hospital," *Journal of Law and Contemporary Problems*, vol. 35 (1970), pp. 817–38.

89. Hertzler, *Horse and Buggy Doctor*.

90. Commission on Hospital Care, *Hospital Care in the United States* (New York: Commonwealth Fund, 1947), pp. 527–59.

91. Lynaugh, "Community Hospitals"; and Robert B. Parks, *Community Health Services for New York City* (New York: Frederick A. Praeger, 1968), pp. 286–88.

92. Davis and Rorem, *Crisis in Hospital Finance*, pp. 141–43.

93. Starr, *Social Transformation*, pp. 166–67; and J. Rogers Hollingsworth, *A Political Economy of Medicine: Great Britain and the United States* (Baltimore: Johns Hopkins University Press, 1986).

94. C. St. Guild, *A Survey of the Medical Facilities in Three Representative Southern Counties* (Chicago: University of Chicago Press, 1932); and W. S. Rankin, "The Small General Hospital," *Hospitals*, vol. 10 (October 1936), pp. 48–52.

95. Steinwald and Neuhauser, "Role of Proprietary Hospital," p. 828.

96. Roemer and Friedman, *Doctors in Hospitals*, p. 144.

97. Lloyd L. Cannedy, "An Historical Analysis of the Viability of For-Profit

Hospitals," *Hospital Progress*, vol. 50 (November 1970), pp. 65–71; and Stein-wald and Neuhauser, "Role of Proprietary Hospital."

98. Committee on Implications of For-Profit Enterprise in Health Care, Institute of Medicine, Bradford H. Gray, ed., *For-Profit Enterprise in Health Care* (Washington, D.C.: National Academy Press, 1986), chap. 3, pp. 47–73. Here-after cited as Gray, *For-Profit Enterprise*.

99. Kenneth Arrow, "Uncertainty and the Welfare Economics of Medical Care," *American Economic Review,* vol. 53 (1963), pp. 941, 950; and Henry B. Hansmann, "The Role of Nonprofit Enterprise," *Yale Law Journal*, vol. 89 (April 1980), pp. 843–44.

100. Mullner et al., "Debt Financing," pp. 18–24.

101. Robert A. Musacchio, Stephen Zuckerman, Lynn E. Jensen, and Larry Freshnock, "Hospital Ownership and the Practice of Medicine: Evi-dence from the Physician's Perspective," in Gray, *For-Profit Enterprise*.

102. Arnold S. Relman, "Investor-owned Hospitals and Health-Care Costs," *New England Journal of Medicine,* vol. 309 (August 11, 1983), pp. 370–72.

103. David Stewart, "The History and Status of Proprietary Hospitals," *Blue Cross Reports*, Research Series 9, March 1973.

104. Ekaterina Siafaca, *Investor-owned Hospitals and Their Role in the Changing U.S. Health Care System* (New York: F & S Press, 1981), p. 105.

105. Ibid.; Gray, *New Health Care*; and Goldsmith, *Can Hospitals Survive?*

106. Montague Brown, "Contract Management: Latest Development in the Trend toward Regionalization of Hospital and Health Services," *Hospital and Health Services Administration* (Winter 1976), pp. 46–67; and Starkweather, *Hospital Mergers in the Making*.

107. Ross Mullner and Jack Hadley, "Interstate Variation in the Growth of Chain-owned Proprietary Hospitals, 1973–1982," *Inquiry,* vol. 21 (Summer 1984), pp. 144–51; and Bays, "Patterns of Hospital Growth."

108. Gwen Kinkead, "Humana's Hard-Sell Hospitals," *Fortune,* November 17, 1980, pp. 68–81; also personal interviews with Humana management and executives of the Federation of American Hospitals.

109. Gray, *New Health Care*, pp. 44–45.

110. National Forum on Hospital and Health Affairs, *A Decade of Implemen-tation* (Durham, N.C.: Duke University, 1975).

111. These observations were made as a result of interviews with ex-ecutives of the Humana Corporation and interviews with physicians affiliated with Humana hospitals. See also Musacchio et al., "Hospital Ownership."

112. Brown, "Contract Management," pp. 40–59; Montague Brown and Howard L. Lewis, *Hospital Management Systems* (Germantown, Md.: Aspen Systems, 1976), pp. 47, 56, 98, 102; and Starkweather, *Hospital Mergers in the Making*.

113. David B. Starkweather, "U.S. Hospitals: Corporate Concentration vs. Local Community Control," *Bulletin of the Institute of Governmental Studies*, vol. 22 (April 1981), p. 5, and *Hospital Mergers in the Making*.

114. Brown, "Contract Management"; and Starkweather, *Hospital Mergers in the Making*.

115. Jay Forrester, *World Dynamics* (Cambridge, Mass.: Wright Allan Press, 1971); and Brown and Lewis, *Hospital Management Systems*, p. 58.

116. Elsworth Smith and Dorothy Cobb, "Are Hospitals Still Sharing?" *Hospitals,* vol. 57 (September 1, 1983), pp. 67–70.

117. Brown, "Contact Management," pp. 52–53.

118. Jack Milburn, "The Small Hospital under Multiple Unit Management," in National Forum on Hospital and Health Affairs, *A Decade of Implementation,* p. 27; and Richard D. Wittrup, "Point of View: The Crisis in Small Hospitals," *Health Care Management Review,* vol. 3 (1978), pp. 55–57.

119. Montague Brown, "Multihospital Systems: Trends, Issues, and Prospects," in Gerald E. Bisbee Jr., ed., *Multihospital Systems: Policy Issues for the Future* (Chicago: Hospital Research and Educational Trust, 1980), pp. 1–21; and Montague Brown and William H. Money, "Implications of Multihospital Management for Catholic Hospitals," *Hospital Progress,* vol. 56 (September 1975), p. 91.

120. Robert A. Derzon et al., "Management Contracts Seen as Largely Resolving Needs," *Hospitals,* vol. 55 (June 16, 1981), pp. 59–62.

121. Thomas G. Rundall and Wendy K. Lambert, "The Private Management of Public Hospitals," *Health Services Research,* vol. 19 (October 1984), pp. 519–44; and William Shonick and Ruth Roemer, *Public Hospitals under Private Management* (Berkeley: University of California Press, 1983), esp. p. 83.

122. Coyne, "Networking"; and Voluntary Hospitals of America, *The Future of America's Health Care* (Dallas: Voluntary Hospitals of America, undated).

123. Montague Brown, "Current Trends in Cooperative Ventures," *Hospitals,* vol. 48 (June 1, 1974), pp. 40–44.

124. Goldsmith, *Can Hospitals Survive?*

125. Starkweather, "U.S. Hospitals."

126. Mullner et al., "Debt Financing"; and Michael D. Hernandez and Arthur J. Henkel, "Need for Capital May Squeeze Freestanding Institutions into Multi-institutional Arrangements," *Hospitals* (March 1, 1982), pp. 75–77.

127. David G. Williamson, Jr., "The Investor-owned Approach," in National Forum on Hospital and Health Affairs, *A Decade of Implementation,* pp. 40–48. These observations are also based on personal interviews with officials of the Federation of American Hospitals.

128. James E. Ludlam and Joy D. Christensen, "Multihospital Arrangements and the Federal Antitrust Laws," in Bisbee, *Multihospital Systems,* pp. 23–61.

129. Starkweather, "U.S. Hospitals"; and Montague Brown, Michael Warner, Paul R. Luehrs, Theodore E. Krueger III, and John N. Hatfield II, "Trends in Multihospital Systems: A Multiyear Comparison," *Health Care Management Review,* vol. 5 (Fall 1980), pp. 9–22.

130. Goldsmith, *Can Hospitals Survive?*

131. Hadley and Feder, "Troubled Hospitals"; Feder, Hadley, and Mullner, "Poor People"; and Feder, Hadley, and Mullner, "Falling through the Cracks."

132. Dan Ermann and Jon Gabel, "Multihospital Systems: Issues and Empirical Findings," *Health Affairs,* vol. 3 (Spring 1984), pp. 50–64; and Sloan, "Property Rights." See also the literature cited in Ermann and Gabel.

3
Comparing the Behavior of Hospitals over Time

As the previous chapter has demonstrated, not only the basic structure of the American hospital system but also the method of financing hospital services has changed substantially during the twentieth century. Although this study has attempted to explain why the number of hospitals in each of the three sectors has fluctuated considerably—public hospitals for some time assuming a much larger role in the provision of beds and more recently a resurgence in the proportion of beds in proprietary hospitals—thus far the discussion has focused very little on how hospitals in the three sectors differ in their behavior.

Although there is widespread familiarity with the generalizations that proprietary hospitals have been skimming the cream among patients and that public hospitals have been dumping grounds for patients undesired elsewhere, such generalizations have long been supported only by impressionistic and episodic accounts, with very little systematic analysis of hospitals' behavior. Even the recent literature is not very conclusive about differences in behavior: Frank Sloan has reported in several studies that voluntary and for-profit hospitals behave very similarly, but Arnold Relman, reviewing the evidence of Pattison and Katz, the Florida Hospital Cost Containment Board, and Lewin and Associates, has reached quite different conclusions.[1]

A historical perspective is very revealing, however. An analysis of the behavior of hospitals in the three sectors during the past fifty years demonstrates that they have become increasingly similar. The differences that persist are small in comparison with the vast differences that existed fifty years ago.

Thus the purpose of this chapter is to discuss the extent to which the behavior of hospitals in the three sectors has varied at various times and to make some headway in understanding why hospitals have become more similar. A major hypothesis underlying this exploration is that since hospitals in the three sectors have increasingly relied on similar sources of funding and capital, had similar levels of funding, and participated in an economy in which regional differences of income and availability of capital have been diminishing, their behavior should be less distinctive.

Of course, hospitals in the three sectors have not become identical. Various forces cause hospitals to vary in their behavior at any one time. They are tied by forces that reflect their past behavior: specific interest groups retain loyalties to individual hospitals; strong prejudices persist about the appropriateness or inappropriateness of proprietary, voluntary, and public hospitals. Such institutional constraints as being part of a chain, having a medical school affiliation, or being managed by a large management company lead to variations in hospitals' behavior, as do their size and their share of local markets. Research has demonstrated that when hospitals, like other organizations, make serious efforts to restructure themselves and to reshape their behavior, it is difficult to alter their staffs and client relationships. In short, their behavior is tied by their past.[2] Thus, even if their sources and levels of funding became identical, some differences in their behavior would be likely to persist.

This chapter focuses primarily on three periods—1935, 1961, and 1979 to the present—although it also discusses the behavior of the three sectors throughout the period since the 1930s. (For a discussion of concepts and data used in this chapter, see the Appendix.)

The year 1935 is chosen for two reasons. First, it is the first year for which there are relatively good systematic data on most hospitals in the three sectors throughout the country. Second, it was a time when the sources of operating revenue and capital varied greatly among the three sectors. Commercial insurance and other third-party payment schemes existed only on a small scale.

Although insurance and other third-party payment schemes had become quite widespread by 1961, considerable variation persisted in sources of funding. Medicare and Medicaid had not yet come into existence. Even so, because the variation in the sources of income had narrowed, the choice of 1961 permits an analysis of whether the variation in behavior had narrowed and how funding changes affect behavior.

By 1979 the sources of funding had converged to a much greater extent. Indeed, by 1979 hospitals were increasingly raising both their income and their capital from very similar sources, especially after the enactment of Medicare and Medicaid in 1965. If convergence in sources of revenue should make hospitals' behavior more similar, their behavior should have been much more similar in 1979 than in 1935. Neither this study nor those cited in it have had data reflecting Medicare reimbursement under diagnosis-related groups (DRGs).

Concepts and Indicators of Hospital Behavior

A vast array of concepts and indicators may be used to compare the behavior of hospitals over time and across sectors. Unfortunately, there is no standardized method of assessing how well hospitals perform the tasks for which they were established. In the absence of data on the outcome of cases for large numbers of hospitals and of any consensus on how to measure the performance of hospitals, this study must rely on more traditional methods of assessing their behavior. Ideally, we would like to compare hospitals in their financial arrangements, technological complexity, case mix, quality of care, number of beds, use, and equality of access by social classes and income groups. For some of these measures, the indicators are much more straightforward than for others. There are no systematic data on sources of revenue and capital for each hospital, but there are sufficient aggregate data to discern the nature of variation in those sources over time.

Measures of costs have a standard meaning in the literature, and relatively good data exist on cost per patient day, cost per patient bed, and cost per patient admission. Data also exist on assets, expenses, and profit margins.

A number of studies have analyzed the facilities and services of American hospitals but have rarely focused on how those have changed over time by sector. Because it is desirable to compare the technological complexity of hospitals and data on facilities and services speak to technological complexity, we also compare facilities and services.

Scholars still wrestle unsuccessfully with the concept of quality of care without reaching a consensus on how to measure it. Even with a consensus, the data for analyzing changes in quality of care would hardly be available. We recognize that at best we can rely on only a few indicators of quality.[3] We thus do not claim to have systematic data that permit us to measure the quality of hospitals directly but rely on input measures that speak indirectly to the quality of care. Specifically, we focus on personnel and on accreditation and affiliation measures.

We also compare the extent to which hospitals are fully occupied and the extent to which their case mix is oriented toward acute care. Finally, we make some effort to compare the accessibility of hospitals in the three sectors to various social classes and income groups.

At different times, because of variations in the available data, it is necessary to use somewhat different indicators of performance. With the passage of time, the indicators have become more numerous and complex. For the earliest time the analysis is confined to aggregate data, but for later times it is more feasible to employ statistical controls in making comparisons. Because data on individual hospitals are not available for 1935, it is often not possible to control for number of beds, for example.

Comparing Hospitals in the Three Sectors, 1935

In 1935 the size of a community very much influenced whether it would have a voluntary or a proprietary hospital.[4] Table 6 demonstrates that as the size of a community increased, so did the proportion of hospitals in the voluntary sector: 39 percent of general hospitals in small cities and about 70 percent in larger cities were in the voluntary sector. As cities increased in size, they had more capital and greater ethnic and religious heterogeneity—two major factors in the rise of voluntary hospitals. Smaller communities had less capital—a factor that fifty years ago gave rise to proprietary hospitals. Almost half the hospitals in communities with populations of fewer than 40,000 were in the proprietary sector.

Although much of the literature about public hospitals has focused on their metropolitan, almshouse antecedents, 40 percent of all public hospitals in 1935 were in cities with fewer than 40,000 residents. Indeed, there seems to have been no systematic relationship between city size and proportion of hospitals in the public sector.

Type of ownership and size of community together exercised a major influence on the size of hospitals in all three sectors. Because a sizable proportion of proprietary hospitals were in small cities and their capital was provided by one or a few entrepreneurs, it is not surprising that the average size of hospitals was smallest in the proprietary sector: 23 beds. In fact, 83 percent of all proprietary hospitals had fewer than 50 beds, 57 percent had fewer than 25 beds, and only 1 percent had more than 150 beds. Voluntary hospitals averaged 92 beds, and public hospitals were largest with an average of 156 beds. Within each major region of the country, the pattern was the same: public hospitals were the largest and proprietary hospitals the smallest.

Their substantially differing sources of income made the hospitals responsive to very different constituencies with varying preferences for hospital behavior. Voluntary nonprofit hospitals derived 71 percent of their operating expenses from patients' fees, public hospitals only 17 percent, and proprietary hospitals 91 percent. In contrast, public hospitals received 81 percent of their operating revenues from

TABLE 6
Public, Voluntary, and Proprietary Hospitals, 1935

	Public Hospitals	Voluntary Hospitals	Proprietary Hospitals	All Hospitals
Average numbers of beds	156	92	23	70
Distribution by number of beds (%)				
Under 25	16.5	11.9	56.7	27.6
25–49	27.6	21.9	26.7	24.2
50–149	29.0	44.9	15.6	33.1
150 and over	26.9	21.3	1.0	15.1
Total	100.0	100.0	100.0	100.0
Community size (%)				
Under 40,000	12.5	39.0	48.5	100.0
40,000–99,999	12.4	57.5	30.1	100.0
100,000–249,000	15.4	61.6	23.0	100.0
250,000 and over	10.9	69.1	20.0	100.0
Source of operating revenue (%)				
Patients	16.7	70.9	91.4	62.4
Taxes	81.0	10.3	4.1	23.8
Endowments	0.5	6.3	0.5	0.0
Gifts	1.8	12.5	4.0	13.8
Total	100.0	100.0	100.0	100.0
Equality of access for social classes and income groups	most accessible	inter-mediate	least accessible	
Rate of occupancy (%)	79	63	45	57
Length of stay (days)	18.3	11.9	9.2	13.1
Assets per bed (dollars)	3,887	5,483	2,486	4,432
Endowment per bed (dollars)	144	1,633	127	1,090
Expenses (dollars)				
Per bed yearly	850	1,198	915	1,073
Per patient day	3.05	5.24	4.44	n.a.
Per patient admission	55.96	65.66	54.83	n.a.
Income per bed, annual (dollars)	850	1,158	960	1,054
Indicators of quality				
Nurses per bed	0.23	0.38	0.26	0.33
Employees per bed	0.63	0.87	0.56	0.77
Employees per 1,000 patients	800	1,400	1,000	n.a.
Accredited by American College of Surgeons (%)	42.9	57.1	14.8	41.1
Value of equipment per bed (dollars)	62.60	76.80	45.00	64.18

n.a. = not available.
Sources: Cited in Appendix.

taxes, proprietary hospitals 4 percent, and voluntary nonprofit hospitals 10 percent. Public and proprietary hospitals received very little revenue from endowments and gifts, but voluntary hospitals received almost 20 percent from those sources. Throughout the country hundreds of voluntary hospitals annually engaged in substantial community fund raising.[5]

Of course, the financing of hospitals varied across the country. In 1934 only 2 percent of the operating revenues of the twelve public hospitals in New York was derived from patients' fees, and in thirty-two nonprofit hospitals in Philadelphia patients paid for only 59 percent of the operating costs. One scholar estimated that communities throughout the country donated from 10 to 40 percent of the operating costs of nonprofit voluntary hospitals.[6]

The sources of revenue did not generally vary with the number of beds except for small public hospitals. Public hospitals with fewer than fifty beds derived almost 60 percent of their revenues from patients, about the same portion as voluntary hospitals of the same size. As a result, small public and voluntary hospitals were more similar in their behavior than other hospitals in the two sectors, for the larger ones derived their revenues from quite different sources.

The 30 percent of revenue that voluntary hospitals received from taxes, endowments, and gifts meant that they were responsive to a more complex constituency than proprietary hospitals, and for this reason they were under greater pressure to provide community-oriented services, such as emergency rooms and teaching facilities. The proprietary sector, because of its dependency on private paying patients, was more constrained by the demands of individual patients. The public sector—much more dependent on the public purse than the two other sectors—provided more community-oriented services than the proprietary sector but, being less dependent on private patients than either the voluntary or the proprietary hospitals, was less oriented toward the amenities demanded by such patients.

Historically, one of the main differences between proprietary hospitals and those in the voluntary and public sectors has been in the degree to which they have provided purely private goods. Of course, most hospitals have provided some combination of private and community services. In general, the source of revenue of hospitals in 1935 influenced the services they provided. Hospitals that received all their revenues from patients' fees were less inclined to provide community-wide services. The less a hospital was under pressure to maximize profits, the greater its opportunity to serve a larger constituency. Hospitals that provided services at less than average costs could do so because they received more revenue from sources other than patients' fees. Of course, hospitals could finance community services from their profits, but the greater the hospital's dependency on grants and gifts, the greater was its ability to produce community services and to serve a larger constituency.

Similarly, variation in the sources of capital for construction induced variability in behavior. Throughout the 1920s and 1930s the major sources of financing for capital expansion of voluntary and public hospitals were philanthropic donations and government taxes.

During the late 1920s almost three quarters of capital for hospital construction came from philanthropy and approximately one quarter from government. The depression changed this pattern dramatically, so that in 1935 approximately 23 percent of all capital came from the voluntary sector and about 73 percent from the public sector. Although local governments occasionally provided some capital for voluntary hospitals, most confined their investment to public hospitals, which derived virtually all their funding from local taxes. Although many new public hospitals were initially financed through the issuance of bonds, the interest and principal were ultimately financed through local taxes. As hospital construction declined during the depression, however, the federal government provided grants, loans, and construction workers for public and voluntary hospital construction under the auspices of the Public Works Agency, the Works Progress Administration, and the Reconstruction Finance Corporation.

The major source of capital for voluntary hospitals during the 1930s was philanthropy, including public subscription drives, donations from wealthy patrons and religious organizations, and community fund raising. Highly publicized fund-raising drives increased the community's interest in the local hospital and encouraged the hospital to be responsive to community needs. In contrast, the proprietary sector was generally funded by a few private practitioners and by patients' fees. Grants from government and philanthropy were small or nonexistent. The proprietary hospital was an adjunct of the private practices of independent physicians and contained the apparatus necessary for their specific practices; as a result, communities did not feel the close attachment to such hospitals that they felt to local voluntary and public hospitals.[7]

The three kinds of hospitals clearly differed in 1935 in the kinds of patients and cases they treated. Proprietary hospitals provided relatively little care to nonpaying patients and specialized almost exclusively in short-term care; about 2 percent of their patients were nonpaying or charity patients. Public sector hospitals served a much higher proportion of nonpaying patients with chronic illnesses. Voluntary hospitals also provided a great deal of charity care although the degree of access by various social classes and income groups varied among regions and within regions by size of hospital. The larger the city and the larger the hospital, the more resources were available for charity patients and the larger the proportion of patients who received charity care.

In a number of large cities, substantial charity care was provided in voluntary and public hospitals in 1935. Approximately three-fourths of all patient days in New York City hospitals were for patients who paid for no part of their care. Of course, charity care in voluntary hospitals was not financed exclusively by the voluntary sector. In New York City one-fourth of the indigent care funded by the public sector was provided by voluntary hospitals.

Because there were more resources for the indigent in the Northeast, the amount of charity work in voluntary hospitals was greater than in less prosperous and less urban areas. Approximately 45 percent of patients in New York City's voluntary hospitals, 30 percent in voluntary hospitals in North and South Carolina, and about 17 percent in Georgia were nonpaying. In a number of midwestern cities with fewer than 50,000 people, voluntary hospitals provided only 10 percent of their services to nonpaying patients.[8]

Even though charity was still widespread in 1935, many people lacked access to hospitals. Throughout the country access to care varied greatly with patients' income. Those with the highest incomes ($10,000 or more) received approximately 25 percent more days of hospital care than those with the lowest incomes (under $1,200). But because those with the lowest incomes frequently had access to free care, they received more days of hospital care than those of middle income ($3,000 to $5,000).[9]

Throughout the country blacks had more difficulty obtaining access to hospitals than any other ethnic group—a phenomenon not limited to the South. Even among New York City's voluntary hospitals, thirteen would not admit blacks to semiprivate rooms, although they would admit them to wards—a pattern that was repeated in large cities across the country.

Another area of considerable variation among the three sectors was in rates of occupancy. Average occupancy was 79 percent in public hospitals, 63 percent in voluntary hospitals, and 45 percent in proprietary hospitals. Occupancy rates were linked to a variety of factors: size of community as well as size of hospital, the number of hospitals in a community, the source of funding, the proportion of patients suffering from chronic illnesses, and the length of stay. In general, the larger the community and the larger the hospital, the greater the funding from the public sector and the larger the proportion of patients with chronic illnesses who stayed for relatively long periods. The longer the average length of stay, the higher the rate of occupancy. The average length of stay was longest in public hospitals (18.3 days), shortest in proprietary hospitals (9.2 days), and intermediate in voluntary hospitals (11.9 days). In some large urban public hospitals, occupancy rates were a serious problem; average occupancy for four of New York City's public general hospitals, for example, exceeded 100 percent.

Even though public hospitals were larger than hospitals in the two other sectors, voluntary hospitals had more assets per bed than either public or proprietary hospitals: 41 percent more than public hospitals and 121 percent more than proprietary hospitals. Given their greater assets, voluntary hospitals predictably had more annual income per bed than public or proprietary hospitals. For-profit hospitals received 13 percent more income per bed than public hospitals.

Of course, expenses per bed were shaped by income per bed. Although the income and expenses of voluntary and proprietary hospitals might diverge for a time, there were constraints on how much they could vary—especially if a hospital encountered deficits. Because legal constraints prevented public hospitals from running deficits, their income and expenses tended to converge. As table 6 demonstrates, voluntary hospitals cost substantially more to operate than public or proprietary hospitals both per patient day and per patient admission. For the nation as a whole, voluntary hospitals ran deficits of 3.5 percent, and proprietary hospitals earned profits of 4.7 percent. Proprietary hospitals earned profits of slightly more than 7 percent except in cities with populations over 250,000, where they often encountered deficits. Quite possibly, it was the competition with voluntary and public hospitals that prevented proprietary hospitals from earning a profit in larger cities.

Public hospitals were not, however, as income and expense figures might suggest, the poor stepchildren of the hospital world. They had 56 percent more assets per bed than proprietary hospitals. This may suggest that public authorities provided initial inputs somewhat more liberally than operating costs. Public hospitals' day-to-day budgets were relatively meager.

Income was tied to various indicators that tap the quality of what occurs in hospitals, however poorly we understand or measure the quality of care. Voluntary hospitals had more personnel of each kind than proprietary or public hospitals. On some measures proprietary hospitals had the fewest staff, on others public hospitals. In New York City, for which there are better data than for other cities for 1935, studies of personnel revealed that more nurses per bed indeed meant better care. Each patient with an acute illness in the wards of voluntary hospitals received approximately 40 percent more nursing time than comparable patients in New York's public hospitals. Similar patterns existed among maternity patients, as well as among those with chronic diseases and other illness. The New York studies concluded that the hospital with fewer personnel had to skimp on routine and indispensable services for body cleanliness and comfort and that many services were improperly delegated to relatively unskilled nursing assistants.[10]

Other indicators of quality, though somewhat crude, also reveal major variations among the three types of ownership. Hospitals did not qualify for interns and residents unless they had the endorsement of the American Medical Association; in 1935 only 11 percent of all hospitals, and virtually no proprietary hospitals, had such approval. Significantly, a somewhat higher percentage of voluntary hospitals than of public hospitals were approved. In the late 1920s, when the American Medical Association considered hundreds of hospitals unworthy of inclusion in its registered list of medical institutions, 67 percent were proprietary hospitals.[11]

Similarly, the American College of Surgeons approved hospitals that met certain standards of performance. In 1935 some 41 percent of general hospitals met the minimum requirements. Again, very few proprietary hospitals gained approval, and a smaller proportion of public hospitals than of voluntary hospitals did so. Low-standard hospitals tended to be very small, and for this reason it was especially difficult for many proprietary hospitals to satisfy certain requirements of the American College of Surgeons and the American Medical Association.

Table 6 also includes the value of medical equipment per bed, a proxy for technological complexity. Voluntary and public hospitals had far more assets in equipment than proprietary hospitals. Since voluntary hospitals were traditionally oriented to acute care, perhaps they had more need to invest in specialized equipment, especially for surgical support. Public hospitals needed less expensive equipment for chronic cases and fewer nurses. Even with the influx of acute cases into public hospitals as a result of the depression of the 1930s, they had fewer such cases than proprietary and voluntary hospitals. Proprietary hospitals had acute-care cases of such a narrow range that they lacked strong incentives to purchase expensive and varied equipment. Because they were smaller, they were less likely to have such basic equipment as clinical laboratories and X-ray service. Among hospitals with fewer than twenty-five beds, however, proprietary hospitals were somewhat better equipped than public or voluntary hospitals.[12]

Many of the indicators for comparing the behavior of 1935 hospitals are systematically related to one another and also to the mixture of cases.

• Public sector hospitals were usually larger and were supported mainly by tax revenues and at a lower level of funding than other hospitals. Payrolls were low (although assets were reasonably high), in part because there were many fewer staff caring for patients. Occupancy rates were quite high because many patients were chronically ill and were nonpaying. Although chronically ill patients required less daily care (and thus less payroll and equipment), they were more often drawn from lower income groups and thus lacked the social status with which to mobilize more money for services.

• Voluntary hospitals, though forced by the depression to move further from their traditions of care for the deserving poor, were nevertheless able to offer higher quality care in part because of their more abundant revenue and assets. Their revenue came mostly from private patients, who were their main users. They chiefly provided acute care, which required more staffing and equipment and thus higher expenses.

• Proprietary hospitals, still very numerous, were small. They were supported almost wholly by patients and thus were able to attract more revenue per patient than hospitals dependent on the public purse. Providing only acute care for more routine ailments, they had short lengths of stay and low occupancy rates. Since they had smaller staffs than voluntary hospitals, their costs were lower, and unlike hospitals in the other two sectors, they earned profits.

Comparing Hospitals in the Three Sectors, 1961

By 1961 the three hospitals sectors had considerably changed vis-à-vis one another from the 1935 pattern. Public hospitals had more than doubled in number, voluntary hospitals had increased substantially, and proprietary hospitals had decreased by 40 percent (from 1,434 in 1935 to 856 in 1960). The total number of general hospitals had increased by one-third and the number of beds by 80 percent. Although the distribution of beds by sector did not precisely track the sectoral changes in number of institutions, the trend was the same for the number of beds as for hospitals (see table 2).

Between 1935 and 1961 several factors did much to transform the American hospital industry. First, the Hill-Burton program made public funding available for hospital construction in many small towns and rural areas, a factor of considerable importance in the increase in public hospitals and decrease in proprietary hospitals in those areas. Second, the rapid growth of private medical insurance helped to increase access to hospital care. Third, rapid changes in the complexity of medical technology enhanced society's belief in the efficacy of hospitals.

A systematic relationship between size of community and distribution of hospitals among the three sectors continued. Although in the 1930s smaller communities tended to have proprietary hospitals, by 1960 they no longer did so. In all bed size classifications, a larger proportion of proprietary hospitals than of public or voluntary hospitals was in large cities. Proprietary hospitals were located predominantly in new and rapidly growing cities, not in the older cities in the eastern regions of the United States. And the smaller the city, the larger the proportion of hospitals that were public.

Because the size of city has a limiting effect on the size of hospitals and a very high proportion of American hospitals were located in small towns and rural areas, the average size of short-term hospitals was still relatively small. Nevertheless, hospitals had become somewhat larger, although proprietary hospitals remained smaller than public and voluntary hospitals. The percentage of proprietary hospitals that had twenty-five or fewer beds had substantially decreased, but 72 percent of proprietary hospitals were still under fifty beds. Approximately 38 percent of the nation's hospitals were under fifty beds, in contrast to 52 percent in 1935. The average hospital sizes were public, 124 beds; voluntary, 139; and proprietary, 45. On the average public hospitals had been diminishing in size, while those in the voluntary and for-profit sectors had increased (see tables 6 and 7).

Perhaps the most important change between 1935 and 1961 was the rapid growth of private medical insurance. In 1935 less than 3 percent of the American population were covered by some form of hospital insurance, but by 1961 approximately two-thirds of the population had some hospital insurance.[13] Yet hospitals still derived their operating revenue from quite different sources. Public hospitals derived 42.0 percent of their revenue from the public sector, voluntary hospitals only 6.5 percent, and proprietary hospitals only 2.1 percent. Proprietary hospitals received virtually all their revenue from patients (97.9 percent), voluntary hospitals 87.1 percent, and public hospitals 58.0 percent. Significantly, philanthropy had become relatively unimportant to operating revenue, providing 6.4 percent in the voluntary sector but virtually nothing in the public and proprietary sectors.[14]

The role of government in financing the operations of nonfederal

TABLE 7
Public, Voluntary, and Proprietary Hospitals, 1961

	Public Hospitals	Voluntary Hospitals	Proprietary Hospitals	All Hospitals
Average number of beds***				
(N = 5,021)	124	139	45	121
Distribution by number of beds (%)[a]				
Under 25	10.0	6.7	32.0	11.4
25–49	33.9	20.0	39.6	26.4
50–99	27.4	25.6	19.5	25.1
100–299	20.9	36.1	8.7	28.2
300 or more	7.8	11.6	0.2	8.9
Total	100.0	100.0	100.0	100.0
Source of revenue(%)[a]				
Consumer	58.0	87.1	97.9	81.6
Government	42.0	6.5	2.1	13.7
Philanthropy	—	6.4	—	4.7
Total	100.0	100.0	100.0	100.0
Equality of access for social classes and income groups				
Discharges not paid by insurance (%)[a]	43.9	26.9	29.8	32.0
Rate of occupancy (%)[a]	72	76	65	74
Length of stay (days)[a]	8.8	7.5	5.8	7.6
Assets per bed (dollars)***				
(N = 4,186)	11,742	13,440	5,571	12,181
Expenses (dollars)				
Per bed yearly[a,]*** (N = 4,521)	5,811.00	7,161.00	6,232.00	6,715.00
Per patient day[a]	33.29	36.04	32.27	34.98
Per admission[a]	281.69	270.06	194.09	267.38
Revenue per bed (dollars)***				
(N = 4,434)	5,608.00	7,342.00	6,671.00	6,846.00
Indicators of quality				
Full-time-equivalent employees per bed[a]	1.6	1.8	1.3	1.7
Residency program approved by American Medical Association (%)***				
(N = 5,042)	11.9	21.6	1.2	16.3
Accreditation, JCAH (%)*** (N = 5,042)	44.6	72.1	21.6	58.1
Technological complexity: facilities and services average				
(maximum = 21)*** (N = 3,973)	10.4	11.9	8.9	11.1

(Notes on next page)

short-term hospitals in the United States was still relatively unimportant. All government sources provided 13.7 percent and philanthropy only 4.7 percent, while consumers paid 81.6 percent.[15]

Although precise data on the extent of insurance payments to hospitals in the three sectors are nonexistent, qualitative data demonstrate substantial variation among the three sectors. Insurance paid for no part of the costs of 44 percent of patients in public hospitals, 27 percent of patients in voluntary hospitals, and 30 percent of patients in proprietary hospitals.[16]

The availability of medical insurance varied greatly with income and age. About 67 percent of the population with annual incomes less than $2,000 and only 15 percent of the population with incomes over $7,000 had no hospital insurance. Some 47 percent of those aged sixty-five to seventy-four and 68 percent of those over seventy-five were without hospital insurance. In sum, millions of low-income and elderly Americans were without any form of third-party coverage for hospital care in 1961, at a time when philanthropic contributions for treating patients were rapidly declining and government contributions, other than for public hospitals, were small. Many poor people simply went without hospital care. Others gravitated to public or voluntary hospitals that provided charity financed by philanthropy or government grants. Of course, hospitals in all three sectors provided charity care through various forms of cross-subsidization, although this was much less common in proprietary than in public and voluntary hospitals.

As the number of public hospitals doubled between 1935 and 1961, many of the smaller ones began to resemble voluntary and proprietary hospitals in being dependent on patients for income and intended to serve the whole community, not just the poor. With the rapid growth of hospital insurance, it became increasingly possible

---

(Notes to table 7)

***Significant at .001 level.

a. Statistical tests cannot be performed because of use of aggregate data.

Sources: Number of beds, yearly expenses per bed, revenue per bed, residency approval by AMA, accreditation by JCAH, and technological complexity from data tape provided by American Hospital Association. Distribution by number of beds, occupancy, length of stay, expenses per patient day and per admission, and full-time-equivalent employees per bed from U.S. Department of Health, Education, and Welfare, Public Health Service, *Medical Care Financing and Utilization*, 1962, data for 1958–1960, tables 105, 108. Source of revenue and discharges not paid by insurance from American Hospital Association, *Hospital Statistics for 1961*.

for public hospitals to attract paying clients, although some large public hospitals remained confined to an indigent clientele, sometimes by statute as well as by custom.

The implications of this change for the behavior of public hospitals were enormous. Although the care of the indigent and chronically ill remained an important responsibility of public hospitals throughout the country, public hospitals became much more heterogeneous. Some, previously subject to the preferences of public policy bodies, were increasingly constrained by the preferences of paying patients, physicians, and insurance companies.

Because of their varied locations, socioeconomic backgrounds of patients, case mixes, sources of funding, and traditions, hospitals in the three sectors also varied in patterns of use. The length of stay for public hospitals (8.8 days) was about 50 percent longer than that for proprietary hospitals (5.8 days) and a sixth longer than for voluntary hospitals. With less variability in case mix, proprietary hospitals had the shortest length of stay.

Because hospitals in the three sectors differed substantially in size, they of course varied in the complexity of their equipment and therefore their assets per bed. Voluntary hospitals, the largest and most complex, had 2.4 times the assets per bed of those in the proprietary sector and about one-seventh more assets per bed than those in the public sector. In 1961 this was still consonant with the circumstances under which proprietary hospitals were created—they were relatively low-cost institutions in rapidly growing areas with shortages of capital or were small hospitals created for the convenience of their doctor-owners.

Significantly, proprietary hospitals were the least costly to operate—whether measured per patient day or per admission—and the voluntary hospitals were generally the most costly. Although no systematic data are available to compare case mixes, scholars have often assumed that the proprietary hospitals were less costly because they engaged in cream skimming.

When controls for size are introduced, the pattern of expenditures by sector becomes more complex. Proprietary hospitals with fewer than 100 beds were 15 to 20 percent more costly per bed than voluntary hospitals and approximately 25 percent more costly than public hospitals of the same size.[17] In general, hospitals of this size provided the same kinds of services, but substantial anecdotal evidence suggests that proprietary hospitals provided more amenities for their patients than voluntary or public hospitals. Public hospitals were less costly per bed than those in the two other sectors. The smaller ones, like those in the voluntary and proprietary sectors, were very dependent on patients' fees for revenue rather than on public subsidies or philanthropy.

By 1961 both proprietary and voluntary hospitals were receiving more revenues than they were spending. The revenues of voluntary hospitals exceeded their expenses by 3 percent, and the surplus of proprietary hospitals was approximately 7 percent. Public hospitals experienced an average loss of about 3 percent. The small public hospitals generally had no losses or profits, but those with more than 300 beds experienced substantial shortfalls. We have no adequate way to measure the relative efficiency of proprietary and voluntary hospitals, since no adequate data exist for 1961 with which it is possible to compare case mixes or outcomes. But if the surplus earned is used as a proxy for efficiency—even if it is a crude proxy—the implications for the efficiency of proprietary hospitals are interesting. Even after allowing for the taxes that proprietary hospitals paid on profits, they still had profit margins approximately twice as great as those earned by voluntary hospitals.

The indicators of quality for hospitals in 1961—as in any other year—are also crude. There were significant differences among the sectors, however, though somewhat less variation than in financial indicators. Nevertheless, there were clear differences in the number of full-time-equivalent staff per bed, the voluntary hospitals having almost 40 percent more staff than proprietary hospitals. The differences between public and voluntary hospitals were smaller. Clear differences were also evident in the hospitals' role as teaching institutions. Although about one-fifth of voluntary hospitals had approved residency programs, only 12 percent of public hospitals and 1 percent of proprietary hospitals did so.

One other indicator deserves comment. The influential Joint Commission on the Accreditation of Hospitals clearly viewed voluntary hospitals as far superior to public hospitals and public hospitals as far superior to proprietary hospitals in granting accreditation. In every size category the proportions of proprietary hospitals accredited showed substantial and statistically significant differences from the proportions of public and voluntary hospitals.

Hospitals in the three sectors varied in the services they provided. Table 7 reports an index of facilities and services, scoring each facility and service provided by hospitals as equal.[18] Of twenty-one facilities and services on which the American Hospital Association collected data, voluntary hospitals offered a third more than proprietary hospitals and almost 15 percent more than public hospitals. In hospitals with fewer than fifty beds, however, the differences among the three sectors were small. Public hospitals with more than 300 beds

101

had 6 to 10 percent more facilities and services than voluntary hospitals, however, suggesting their more diverse constituency.

Differences from sector to sector in basic facilities and services were small. Larger hospitals in each sector offered a broader array than smaller ones, although in all sectors proprietary hospitals offered more restrictive facilities and services.

To sum up the pattern in 1961:

• Hospitals varied substantially in the size of the community in which they existed, and their size varied substantially from one sector to another. The proprietary sector had the smallest hospitals, more frequently located in large urban settings than either public or voluntary hospitals. Consistently with their previous history, however, proprietary hospitals existed primarily in rapidly growing areas where public and voluntary hospitals had not adequately responded to the demand for more beds.

• In access to care, proprietary hospitals remained the most inegalitarian and public hospitals the most egalitarian, especially in large cities.

• Public hospitals had the longest length of stay, proprietary hospitals the shortest—most likely reflecting differences in case mixes.

• Costs per patient day were somewhat higher and costs per admission approximately 40 percent higher in public and voluntary hospitals than in proprietary hospitals. At the same time, profits in proprietary hospitals were at least double those in voluntary hospitals, even after taxes.

• The three sectors also varied substantially in their external accrediting ratings, the extent to which they were involved in training residents and interns, and their array of facilities and services. On all three of these indicators, the differences among the three sectors were statistically significant.

Comparing Hospitals in the Three Sectors, 1979

By 1979 the community hospital sector had expanded vastly, not so much in numbers of institutions as in beds. Bed capacity in acute-care hospitals was nearly 1 million. The distribution of beds among sectors had changed somewhat since 1961. Public hospitals accounted for a somewhat larger percentage of institutions but a smaller percentage of beds. Proprietary hospitals constituted a smaller percentage of institutions but nevertheless had a larger and increasing percentage of beds. The proportion of voluntary hospitals remained more stable (see table 2).

The community sites of hospitals in the three sectors varied less than in the early 1960s. Public hospitals, however, many having been created with the assistance of Hill-Burton funding, continued to be found much more commonly in small towns and rural areas. In the 1980s, when the Health Care Financing Administration identified over 300 hospitals as "sole providers" of services for sizable geographical areas, only a handful of proprietary hospitals were on the list.[19] Proprietary hospitals had moved very far from their original roles as the only providers of services in many communities, but they continued to be located more frequently in larger cities than hospitals in the other two sectors, although voluntary hospitals were close behind.

Even so, by the late 1970s proprietary hospitals had become somewhat less metropolitan than in the 1960s, in part because they had begun to move aggressively into fast-growing secondary cities, and they were located in metropolitan areas only in certain parts of the country. Proprietary chains were usually located in states with few mandatory rate control programs, in areas with low Medicaid and indigent patient loads, and in areas where Blue Cross reimbursed on the basis of charges. In contrast with voluntary and public hospitals, which were located in substantial numbers in all regions and in areas with varying regulatory environments, those in the proprietary sector continued to have much more flexibility and discretion about location.[20] There is still some disagreement about the consequences of the location of for-profit hospitals, some scholars saying that they are located in counties no less poor than other hospital locations.[21] Most scholars, however, believe that they are sited in somewhat richer communities and that such locational choices have indirect effects in creaming, or selecting better-paying clients.

The average hospital had grown considerably larger with the passage of years, to 169 beds. Although the evidence on economies of scale continues to be mixed, many analysts believe that 300-bed hospitals can function more efficiently than those of other sizes.[22] If so, the average American short-term hospital, with 169 beds, was still far too small. Average bed size by sector continued to vary greatly. The average in public hospitals was 116 beds, in voluntary hospitals 210, and in proprietary hospitals 115. Although public and proprietary hospitals were of similar size, public hospitals were much less homogeneous than proprietary hospitals (see table 8).[23] There were still many small hospitals, especially in the public sector. Almost 70 percent of all public hospitals had fewer than 100 beds, in contrast to 50 percent of proprietary hospitals and 35 percent of voluntary hospitals. Significantly, proprietary hospitals were no longer deviant in size, as they had been before the introduction of Medicare and Medi-

TABLE 8
Public, Voluntary, and Proprietary Hospitals, 1979

	Public Hospitals	Voluntary Hospitals	Proprietary Hospitals	All Hospitals
Average number of beds***	116	210	115	169
Distribution by number of beds (%)[a]				
Under 25	7.9	2.9	6.9	4.9
25–49	29.3	12.2	19.3	18.4
50–99	31.8	20.5	26.1	24.7
100–299	22.9	40.7	42.2	35.5
300 or more	8.1	23.7	5.5	16.5
Total	100.0	100.0	100.0	100.0
Source of revenue (%)[a]				
Medicare	34	34	33	33.7
Medicaid	11	7	7	7.5
Blue Cross	n.a.	n.a.	n.a.	16.3
Other insurance	n.a.	n.a.	n.a.	15.6
Other sources	n.a.	n.a.	n.a.	26.9
Total				100.0
Equality of access for social classes and income groups (ratio of uncompensated charges to total charges)[a,b]				
Teaching hospitals	2.77	0.90	0.65	—
Nonteaching hospitals	1.41	0.79		
Rate of occupancy (%)[a]	69.1	76.5	63.9	73.8
Length of stay (days)*** (N = 5,750)	7.7	8.0	6.6	7.7
Assets per bed (dollars)[a]	43,437.00	48,883.00	40,375.00	47,010.00
Expenses (dollars)[a]				
Per bed yearly	62,573.00	69,492.00	57,840.00	67,009.00
Per patient day	205.10	217.93	225.87	215.75
Per patient admission	1,524.24	1,681.70	1,477.33	1,631.16
Revenue per inpatient day (dollars)[a]	n.a.	253.67	n.a.	249.84
Indicators of quality (N = 5,750)				
Full-time-equivalent employees per bed***	2.7	2.9	2.1	2.8
Residency program approved by American Medical Association (%)***	9.5	21.5	1.2	15.2

TABLE 8 (continued)

	Public Hospitals	Voluntary Hospitals	Proprietary Hospitals	All Hospitals
Accreditation by Joint Commission on Accreditation of Hospitals (%)***	60.6	82.5	71.5	74.3
Technological complexity: facilities and services average (maximum = 43)*** (N = 5,140)	9.6	14.4	10.3	12.5

***Significant at .001 level.
n.a. = not available.
a. Tests of significance could not be performed because of use of aggregate data.
b. The figures are the ratio of the share of uncompensated care charges to total share of charges, nationwide. If a type of hospital accounted for 53.1 percent of charges nationwide but provided 41.7 percent of uncompensated care nationwide (as did voluntary nonteaching hospitals), the ratio would be 0.79.
SOURCES: Average number of beds, length of stay, indicators of quality, and technological complexity from data tape for 1979 provided by American Hospital Association. Distribution by number of beds, rate of occupancy, expenses, and revenue per inpatient day from American Hospital Association, *Hospital Statistics for 1979*. Source of revenue from Edward R. Becker and Frank A. Sloan, "Hospital Ownership and Performance," *Economic Inquiry*, vol. 23 (January 1985), pp. 21–36. Equality-of-access ratio computed from 1982 data presented by Frank A. Sloan, Joseph Valvona, and Ross Mullner, "Identifying the Issues: A Statistical Profile," in Frank A. Sloan, James Blumstein, and James Perrin, eds., *Uncompensated Hospital Care: Defining Rights and Assigning Responsibilities* (Baltimore: Johns Hopkins University Press, 1985), pp. 16–53. Assets per bed from American Hospital Association, *Hospital Statistics for 1976*.

caid. And as the size of voluntary hospitals began to converge with that of public and proprietary hospitals, so did their behavior.

Between 1961 and 1979 the introduction of Medicare and Medicaid fundamentally changed the sources of revenue of short-term general hospitals. By 1979, 33.7 percent of hospital revenue was derived from Medicare and 7.5 percent from Medicaid. Blue Cross paid 16.3 percent and other insurance 15.6 percent. The remainder, except for self-paying patients, was largely paid by other governmental programs, such as Workers' Compensation.[24] The variation in sources of funding among the three sectors had narrowed substantially since the introduction of Medicare and Medicaid. No longer, as in the early part of the century, were public hospitals alone in deriving much of their funding from the public sector while the proprietary sector received most of its funding from paying patients and the voluntary sector a substantial portion from philanthropy and local governments.

The large proportion of Americans whose hospital care was financed through medical insurance had considerable discretion in choosing a hospital with the understanding that the third-party payer would compensate the hospital for a proportion of the costs. This reimbursement system encouraged hospitals to compete with one another for patients and to become more alike in their facilities and services.

The American Hospital Association's reimbursement survey for 1979 found that proprietary and voluntary hospitals received 7 percent of their operating revenues from Medicaid and public hospitals 11 percent. All three received approximately one-third of their revenue from Medicare. Certainly in dependence on Medicare and Medicaid voluntary and proprietary hospitals were much alike.[25]

Moreover, most voluntary and proprietary hospitals had become very similar in their willingness to treat patients freely. In metropolitan areas voluntary hospitals had bad debt and charity care amounting to 3.7 percent of total hospital charges; the corresponding percentage was 3 percent for proprietary hospitals and 8.6 percent for public hospitals. In nonmetropolitan areas, however, the percentages were 4 percent for voluntary hospitals, 5.3 percent for public hospitals, and 4.2 percent for proprietary hospitals. In the nation as a whole public hospitals provided almost twice their proportionate share of free care.

These data, combined with data on the Medicaid and Medicare patients treated by voluntary and proprietary hospitals, raise important questions about the extent to which proprietary hospitals were engaging in cream skimming on the scale that many observers had hitherto believed. Office for Civil Rights data for two weeks in 1981 corroborate the impression that for-profit and voluntary hospitals exhibited small differences in their provision of care to the uninsured.[26] Defending the behavior of investor-owned hospitals, some scholars have suggested that since for-profit hospitals pay taxes, they have already met their social obligations and do not have further responsibilities to provide charity care.[27]

Arnold Relman has suggested that in discussing cream skimming, we should be sensitive to the idea that locational choices themselves are a form of cream skimming. Other critics of the amount of free care provided by for-profit hospitals question the common practice of combining bad debt and charity care in discussing charity care. They contend that for-profit hospitals may be providing their free care involuntarily, by reclassifying their bad debts as free care, whereas voluntary hospitals are voluntarily giving charitable care. Unfortunately, because even the best available data for the nation as a whole generally do not permit dividing bad debt from charity care, there is no firm evidence with which to refute or substantiate such opinions.[28]

There is evidence, however, that in some states in which for-profit hospitals constitute a large share of the market, they provide less charity care than voluntary hospitals. California data do not support these findings, which are based on Florida, Tennessee, Texas, and Virginia.[29]

In the 100 largest cities in 1980 the large public hospitals provided more than their share of free care. Nonprofit hospitals provided approximately 20 percent less than their share. Throughout the country a relatively few hospitals in the three sectors provided most of the free care for the poor. In California Pattison and Katz found charity as a percentage of net revenue approximately zero for all three kinds of hospitals. In short, there was still unequal access to hospitals for the country as a whole, public hospitals continuing to be somewhat more accessible. Although some voluntary hospitals were more accessible to the poor in the nation's 100 largest cities than proprietary hospitals, for the nation as a whole there appeared to be only small differences between voluntary and proprietary hospitals in access to care.[30]

The poor continued to have serious difficulty in obtaining access to hospitals. In 1979 approximately 17 million people below 150 percent of the poverty-line income had inadequate medical insurance, and a 1982 survey found that 15 percent of families without hospital insurance needed care during the year but did not receive it. The Institute of Medicine estimated in 1985 that 35 million people were without hospital insurance.[31]

As variation in sources of revenue and in patients narrowed among the three sectors, so did rates of occupancy and lengths of stay. The traditional pattern of high occupancy and long stays in public hospitals was no longer so pronounced. In fact, in 1979 public hospitals had lower occupancy rates and shorter lengths of stay than voluntary hospitals, mainly because of the large proportion of public hospitals in small towns and rural areas and their mixture of cases.

The issue of length of stay speaks to the allegation that investor-owned hospitals have continued to have shorter stays because they systematically select the most profitable patients. Most studies of cream skimming and length of stay in hospitals have relied on small samples, usually in a particular region, but one study, based on hospital admissions throughout the country in 1976, demonstrated that after controlling for case mix and various hospital characteristics, there were no statistically significant differences in length of stay between voluntary and for-profit hospitals. Voluntary hospitals, however, had somewhat older patients and more patients with cancer. Whether the two types of hospitals had somewhat different patients because of cream skimming, location, or a combination of these or other reasons remains a question high on the research agenda, although statewide studies using more recent data indicate that proprietary and voluntary hospitals did not treat significantly different kinds of cases.[32]

The various indicators of quality of care remain crude. Even if scholars still do not have adequate methods and data with which to measure quality of care, a variety of indicators speak in some fashion to the issue of quality: various input measures, the characteristics of hospital staff and physicians, accreditation by major professional associations, an accredited residency program, and medical school affiliation. And even if the reader disagrees that these are measures of quality, we nevertheless believe it useful to compare hospitals in terms of these indicators.

Significantly, voluntary hospitals had 20 percent more full-time professional staff per bed (including nurses as well as doctors) than proprietary hospitals in 1979. The characteristics of doctors on the staffs of voluntary and proprietary hospitals were much more similar when hospitals were matched by length of stay of patients, kind of service, size of hospital, and geographic location.[33] Indeed, one of the issues of great interest in comparing the quality of medical service in hospitals has been the characteristics of their staff physicians. Several recent studies have concluded that investor-owned hospitals accept a slightly higher percentage of medical staff applicants, have slightly more physicians per bed, have slightly higher rates of board certification among the medical specialties and somewhat lower rates among the surgical specialties, including obstetrics and gynecology, have fewer specialists, and have physicians with fewer years of hospital affiliation.[34]

Some differences in quality between the medical staffs of voluntary and for-profit hospitals are explained largely by system size, hospital size, teaching activity, region of the country, and size of the community.[35] Once these factors are controlled, voluntary and for-profit hospitals are quite similar in staff size and composition and criteria for review of privileges.[36]

108

Another approach to quality considers how physicians view for-profit and nonprofit hospitals and whether their personal experiences with for-profit hospitals influence their opinions about aspects of hospital quality. The 1984 American Medical Association survey of physicians' opinions found that 50 percent of doctors thought that nonprofit hospitals provided the same quality of care as for-profit hospitals; 37 percent thought that physicians had the same amount of clinical discretion at a for-profit hospital (28 percent thought they had less discretion, 9 percent that they had more). Asked whether they would prefer to practice in a nonprofit or a for-profit setting if medical staff privileges, compensation arrangements, and work conditions were the same, 51 percent said they had no preference, and 42 percent preferred the nonprofit setting. On these three indicators—perceptions about quality of care, clinical discretion, and preference for practice—doctors who had reported some involvement with for-profit hospitals had somewhat more favorable attitudes toward them than those who had had no such contact.[37]

Several studies have suggested a link between quality of care and doctors' involvement in hospital governance. Recent studies show that more doctors are found on the governing boards of for-profit than of voluntary hospitals, that doctors in for-profit hospitals are more likely than those in voluntary hospitals to report that administrators are responsive to the needs of staff physicians, and that the chairperson of a hospital governing board is far more likely to be a physician in an investor-owned hospital than in other kinds of hospitals.[38]

On other issues that speak to quality, there was less similarity. In 1979 the three sectors varied substantially in their educational programs. Only 1 percent of proprietary hospitals had residency programs approved by the American Medical Association, in contrast to 22 percent of voluntary hospitals and 10 percent of public hospitals. Moreover, slightly less than 1 percent of proprietary hospitals were affiliated with medical schools, while the corresponding numbers were 17 percent for voluntary hospitals and 8 percent for public hospitals. A larger percentage of proprietary hospitals than of public hospitals were approved in 1979 by the Joint Commission on Accreditation of Hospitals—a result of the large number of small public hospitals. Only 29 percent of the 665 public hospitals with fewer than fifty beds were accredited. More recent data reveal that investor-owned system hospitals were more likely than any other kind of hospital to be accredited.[39]

Since 1935 the differences in technological complexity of hospitals in the three sectors had narrowed considerably. Voluntary hospitals provided the most facilities and services, followed by proprietary hospitals and then by public hospitals. The variation in facilities and services was closely related to variation in size. In each sector technological complexity—that is, facilities and services—increased with the size of hospitals. Hardly any variation in technological complexity existed in hospitals with fewer than 200 beds, but proprietary hospitals had fewer facilities and services than public and voluntary hospitals as size increased beyond 200 beds.

Virtually all hospitals (regardless of size and sector) had such basic services as postoperative recovery rooms, pharmacies, respiratory therapy facilities, and emergency rooms, and most had physical therapy facilities and blood banks. Differences in more expensive and novel facilities and services were more distinct. Voluntary hospitals were much more likely to have facilities requiring complex equipment and special staffing (cardiac catheterization equipment and CT scanners), programs responding to special needs (home care, organ banks, premature nurseries, genetic counseling), and socially controversial programs (alcohol and chemical dependency programs). The decisions of voluntary hospitals were probably influenced in part by their larger size. With more beds, they were able to finance a broader array of services, especially services using more expensive technologies.

Large urban public hospitals assumed a greater role in providing facilities and services for lower-income groups. Moreover, burn centers and trauma centers were much more common in public hospitals. But innovative programming not addressed to lower-income groups was most frequently offered in voluntary hospitals.

Investor-owned proprietary hospitals frequently made special efforts to provide amenities or services unique in their communities. Rather than emphasizing a vast array of services, they often provided custom-tailored delivery of services or made efforts to address specific market niches.

One study of Florida investor-owned and voluntary hospitals confronted the question whether proprietary and voluntary hospitals differed in the array of unprofitable services they offered. The authors found no significant differences in the degree to which the two kinds of hospitals offered profitable and unprofitable services. This kind of analysis has not been carried out with national data.[40]

Economists have long theorized that for-profit hospitals should be less expensive than those in which the profit or surplus incentive is absent. The questions whether their theories can be supported by empirical studies and what kinds of studies are most appropriate have filled the scholarly and policy literature for the past several years, and some form of consensus is only now emerging. Values have come into

110

play as scholars and doctors have written about the issues of cost and efficiency, and this area of inquiry has generated a great deal of heat. Probably the issue that has been of greatest interest is whether for-profit hospitals in chains differ in their financial performance from voluntary hospitals, that is, whether so-called corporate medicine costs more or less.

Studies have usually focused on four indicators: (1) the cost or expense to the hospital for taking care of the patient per day or per admission, (2) the charge or price the hospital levies for care per day or per admission, (3) the markup the hospital uses in pricing services, and (4) the amount of profit or surplus made by the hospital. Other comparisons are used more occasionally, especially the ratio of assets to revenues and the net community "contribution."

Comparisons of these four indicators are made for voluntary, for-profit, and public hospitals in table 8, which indicates that expenses per patient admission are highest in voluntary hospitals and lowest in proprietary hospitals. Voluntary hospitals spend 13.8 percent more per admission than for-profit hospitals. For-profit hospitals are 3.6 percent more expensive per day than voluntary hospitals, and public hospitals are least expensive. These are, of course, simply raw figures, without controls for other characteristics.

Several scholars, however, have introduced a great deal more complexity into the analysis, either by pairing hospitals on a large number of characteristics or by using national, regional, or large state samples with statistical controls to standardize for variables such as bed size and case mix. Other controls that have been used are rural-urban location, scale of teaching activity, adjustments for outliers, standardization of accounting procedures, and membership in a chain or system.

The problem of comparing costs among the three kinds of hospitals is further complicated by the existence in each kind of both free-standing hospitals and hospitals in chains. Because considerable evidence suggests that being part of a chain influences the behavior of hospitals, it is important to differentiate hospitals that are in chains from those that are not and, among hospitals in chains, those that have recently joined from those that have long been in a chain. Since a newly acquired hospital often has considerable new expense, it frequently takes several years to become cost effective. For this reason, it is useful for an analysis of hospital costs to be sensitive to differences between new and old chains.

Given this panoply of variables and the considerable divergence in research questions, it is not surprising that various studies have come to somewhat different conclusions. To some extent this may be

111

attributable to the different universes of hospitals studied, as well as to the variables included and the variation in time periods. More and more scholars have moved to quite large, even national, samples, obtained data for several years, and included a wide range of variables sensitive to location, case mix, and the like. A further complication in understanding the behavior of hospitals, however, is that several studies have excluded public hospitals from their analysis.

One finding seems clear. For-profit chain hospitals do not cost less per day or per case than voluntary hospitals (regardless of the number of variables controlled in the analysis). Their expenses in caring for patients are no lower; their charges are no lower. Several studies report quite the reverse—that for-profit chain hospitals have higher expenses per patient and per admission and that they charge patients more for care. The differences are sometimes, but not uniformly, statistically significant.

Three recent studies on cost comparison are based on national data sets, although one of them did not include public hospitals. Their findings are fairly close, though not in total accord. Watt and his colleagues, using 1980 data for 561 hospitals and twenty-eight control variables, report that patient care expenses and total operating expenses per case were much the same for investor-owned and independent for-profit hospitals, government hospitals, and both system and independent voluntary hospitals. Analyzing more than 1,600 hospitals with data for six years and using approximately thirty control variables, Coelen found that total expenses per adjusted discharge were higher for proprietary chains than for independent voluntary hospitals but that both independent proprietary and chain voluntary hospitals had lower expenses than independent voluntary hospitals. Becker and Sloan, using 1979 data on 1,645 hospitals and controlling for a large number of independent variables, found that independent for-profit hospitals were more expensive per day than other independent hospitals but were less costly per admission. For-profit chain hospitals, per day and per admission, were more costly than independent voluntary hospitals.[41]

One of these data sets, drawn for 1979 and therefore complementary to the analysis presented in this section, also addresses the effects on cost of being in a chain or system and of being an old or a new chain member (see table 9).[42] These data also illustrate just how complex the analysis can be. The study controls for variables related to chain status, teaching status, mixture of third-party payers, case mix, bed size, age of hospital, wages in the hospital, per capita income of patients in the hospitals' immediate environment, and region. With these variables controlled for, independent proprietary

112

TABLE 9

COMPARISON OF COSTS AND PROFITS OF VOLUNTARY
AND OTHER HOSPITALS, 1979

	Independent	Old Chain[a]	New Chain
Voluntary			
Cost per day[b]	—	2	2
Cost per case[b]	—	2	1
Profit[c]	—	0	−1
Public			
Cost per day[b]	2	2	−6
Cost per case[b]	0	−2	11***
Profit[c]	−1**	−5**	−1
Proprietary			
Cost per day[b]	9*	15***	10***
Cost per case[b]	−5	6	12***
Profit[c]	−1	−2	0

NOTE: Comparisons are in terms of percentage of difference from the reference category, independent voluntary hospitals.
* Significant at .10 level.
** Significant at .05 level.
***Significant at .01 level.
a. "Old" means six years of affiliation for voluntary and public hospitals, four years for proprietary hospitals.
b. Cost figures per patient day and per case are adjusted.
c. Profit refers to the ratio of total revenue to total cost.
SOURCE: Derived from Edmund R. Becker and Frank A. Sloan, "Hospital Ownership and Performance," Economic Inquiry, vol. 23 (January 1985), pp. 28–29. In carrying out their analysis, Becker and Sloan used the following control variables: teaching status, mix of third-party payers, case mix, number of beds, age, patient's per capita income, hospital wages, and region.

hospitals were more costly than independent hospitals in the public and voluntary sectors in cost per adjusted patient day but less costly per adjusted admission. Costs of independent public and voluntary hospitals were virtually identical per day and per admission.

The results were quite different for hospitals in chains. Proprietary hospitals, whether new or old affiliates of a chain, were 10 to 15 percent more costly per adjusted patient day than independent voluntary hospitals and were more expensive than hospitals in voluntary or public chains, with either old or new affliations. Similarly, both kinds of proprietary chain hospitals were more expensive in total costs per adjusted admission than either kind of voluntary chain hospital. Surprisingly, the costs per case of public and proprietary hospitals newly joined to chains were similar even though the average length of stay was longer in the public hospitals.

As the table demonstrates, some of these findings are statistically significant, and others are not. The findings that proprietary hospitals new in chains are substantially more expensive per case and per day than free-standing voluntary hospitals are statistically significant.[43]

Herzlinger's study of for-profit and nonprofit chain hospitals from 1977 to 1981 takes into account the public subsidies each form of ownership enjoys.[44] This approach has also been used by Frank Sloan.[45] Herzlinger's findings are that, given the greater subsidies nonprofit chain hospitals obtain, their costs make them an inefficient means of delivering services. Sloan's work, with different kinds of adjustments for subsidies and a different universe, shows more similarity of behavior among hospitals of different ownership.

Other studies using subnational or regional data add to the complexity of the findings. Several of them report that costs are higher in for-profit hospitals,[46] others that costs are much the same.[47]

To generalize from these studies, so varied in the adjustments made to the data and in the focus of investigation, is somewhat complicated. It seems appropriate to conclude, however, that for-profit hospitals do not care for patients more cheaply or economically than voluntary hospitals. The picture for public hospitals is slightly less clear because of their exclusion from several major studies, but the existing studies find public hospitals the least costly.

Several studies have drawn attention to the essential similarity in billable charges for basic services among different kinds of hospitals. But ancillary charges in for-profit hospitals, especially those in chains, are considerably higher than in voluntary and public hospitals. Although these studies are based on different periods and different samples, a good bit of evidence seems to show that overall charges are indeed higher in for-profit chain hospitals. Even though they charge more, the difference is the equivalent of less than one-half of 1 percent of the nation's medical costs.[48]

Profitability among hospitals is a burning issue, just like costs and charges. The conclusions, not unexpectedly, are mixed. In general, studies that have found that costs and charges vary little with ownership type also report that profit differences are small. In reviewing these studies, it is useful to keep in mind that in the past few years hospitals on the average are reporting increasing positive margins. Those positive margins—surpluses or profits as they might equally well be called—have caused a recent committee on the study of the for-profit health sector to suggest that the term "nonprofit" is obsolete.

114

The three studies based on national data also examine profitability among hospitals by ownership type. Becker and Sloan report virtually no differences in profitability between voluntary and for-profit hospitals, whether in chains or not. Public hospitals had the most negative profit pattern. Watt and others, however, report that investor-owned systems and independent for-profit hospitals were more profitable than voluntary hospitals (whether in a system or free-standing) or government hospitals. Coelen's study indicates slightly higher profits for the for-profit hospitals (both chain and independent) than for independent voluntary hospitals. Of these three studies, the one by Watt and others shows the most difference in financial behavior.[49] Other studies have drawn attention to the ability of the for-profit sector to defer a substantial percentage of the taxes owed on profits and thereby retain a greater share of profits than financial statements and accounting sheets may suggest.[50]

Several regional studies, using somewhat different methods, have had rather contradictory findings about the profitability of hospitals. For a sample of Florida hospitals Sloan and Vraciu found the after-tax margin similar for nonprofit and for-profit hospitals, although Lewin and others found proprietary hospitals to have higher profit margins than voluntary hospitals. In a sample of California hospitals, Pattison and Katz found surprisingly that the net income of proprietary hospitals—whether part of a chain or independent—was substantially less than that of voluntary hospitals, measured per patient day or per admission.[51]

Undoubtedly, the profit margins of various kinds of hospitals varied from locale to locale. Voluntary hospitals that provided a low percentage of their total care to the poor in 1980 had large profit margins, while those that provided a relatively high percentage of their total care to the poor experienced substantial deficits. In 1980 voluntary and public hospitals for the nation as a whole were averaging a profit margin of approximately 3 percent. Because almost one-fourth of these hospitals operated at a loss, however, the issue of deficits was very serious, especially among the large urban hospitals that provided substantial care to the poor.[52]

The following were a few of the more salient patterns in 1979:

• A higher proportion of public hospitals than of proprietary and voluntary hospitals were in small communities. Largely because of Medicare, the size of proprietary hospitals had increased substantially.

• Because all three sectors received revenues from similar sources, the facilities and services of proprietary hospitals no longer deviated substantially from those in the public and voluntary sectors.

• After controlling for case mix and various hospital characteristics, there were no statistically significant differences in length of stay between voluntary and proprietary hospitals, although they did differ somewhat in the patients they treated.

• In the nation as a whole voluntary and proprietary hospitals provided comparable but relatively small amounts of free care, and public hospitals provided more than their proportionate share.

• Costs for hospital care were lowest in public hospitals. Although costs in voluntary and for-profit hospitals appeared similar in many studies, there is enough evidence to suggest rather strongly that for-profit hospital costs per case were higher.

• Overall, costs in chain-affiliated hospitals were higher than costs in free-standing hospitals. Costs in proprietary chains were higher than those in voluntary chains, and costs in hospitals newly affiliated to chains were higher than in hospitals that had been in chains longer.

• Charges for hospital care were lower in public hospitals than in voluntary or for-profit hospitals. Most studies agree that charges were higher in for-profit hospitals than in voluntary hospitals, although this question remains in lively dispute.

• Profits of for-profit hospitals, especially those in chains, were greater than profits in voluntary hospitals, whether chain or independent. Public hospitals were least likely to report profits.

Concluding Observations

In recent years American society has felt considerable concern about how nonprofit hospitals—whether public or voluntary—behave in relation to proprietary hospitals. Of course, many years ago hospitals in the three sectors behaved very differently from one another. Proprietary hospitals long encountered a lack of legitimacy. Popular views of the contemporary behavior of hospitals in the three sectors have not yet adjusted to reality. Clearly, hospitals in the three sectors do differ somewhat in their behavior, but they have become increasingly similar.

The behavior of the three kinds of hospitals varied considerably in 1935. As table 10 demonstrates, however, the variation has narrowed substantially since then in size of hospital, percentage of hospitals accredited by the major professional associations, length of stay, rate of occupancy, full-time-equivalent staff per bed, technological complexity, costs per bed, and assets per bed. Hospitals are much more alike in the kinds of patients they treat and in the care they provide. Differences from sector to sector are small on financial indicators, occupancy, and length of stay. Seemingly, as variation in case

116

TABLE 10

	Public Hospitals	Voluntary Hospitals	Proprietary Hospitals	Range
Size				
1935	2.23	1.31	0.33	1.90
1961	1.02	1.15	0.37	0.78
1979	0.69	1.23	0.69	0.54
Occupancy				
1935	1.39	1.11	0.79	0.60
1961	0.97	1.02	0.88	0.14
1979	0.94	1.04	0.87	0.17
Length of stay				
1935	1.40	0.91	0.70	0.70
1961	1.16	0.99	0.86	0.30
1979	0.97	1.01	0.87	0.14
Assets per bed				
1935	0.88	1.24	0.56	0.68
1961	0.88	1.10	0.39	0.71
1979	0.92	1.04	0.86	0.18
Expenses per bed				
1935	0.79	1.12	0.85	0.33
1961	0.88	1.05	0.84	0.21
1979	0.93	1.04	0.86	0.18
Expenses per day				
1961	0.95	1.03	0.92	0.11
1979	0.95	1.01	1.05	0.10
Expenses per admission				
1961	1.05	1.01	0.73	0.32
1979	0.93	1.03	0.91	0.12
Quality				
Full-time-equivalent employees per bed				
1935	0.82	1.13	0.73	0.40
1961	0.94	1.06	0.76	0.30
1979	0.96	1.04	0.75	0.29
Accreditation				
1935[a]	1.04	1.39	0.36	1.03
1961[b]	0.77	1.24	0.37	0.87
1979[b]	0.82	1.11	0.96	0.29
Technological complexity				
1935[c]	0.98	1.20	0.70	0.50
1961[d]	0.94	1.07	0.80	0.27
1979[d]	0.77	1.15	0.82	0.38

(Notes on next page)

117

mix has narrowed, so has variation in costs per case and costs per admission.

Differences among sectors remain wider on staffing, accreditation by the Joint Commission on Hospitals, the incidence of residence programs approved by the American Medical Association, and technological complexity. Of course, differences in size remain substantial—indeed larger than any other differences. Large voluntary hospitals, however convergent in financial arrangements, occupancy, and case mix, still provide more complex services that require more personnel.

Why has the behavior of the three kinds of hospitals become more alike in a number of major ways? A couple of considerations must be kept in mind. First, because of the increased belief in the efficaciousness of medical technology, there is less variation in the demand for medical services. Doctors throughout the country have undergone similar training and expect hospitals to be comparable. Moreover, pressures from the accrediting associations have encouraged standardization within hospitals throughout the country.

Of far greater importance in explaining increased similarity, however, is the change in the sources of funding. In the early part of the century public hospitals obtained much of their funding from the public sector, voluntary hospitals from gifts and donations, and proprietary hospitals from paying patients. When they received their funding from distinct sources, they were responsive to very different constituencies with different preferences. Over time, however, the sources of revenue have converged, and the behavior of hospitals has also converged, as reliance on similar funding sources has made hospitals increasingly responsive to the same constituencies. After learning to respond to insurance companies and Blue Cross plans, hospitals learned to adapt to state and federal funding sources. By 1983, with approximately 50 percent of revenue for each sector coming from Medicare and Medicaid, the role of public authorities in funding hospital care was still more important.[53]

(Notes to table 10)

NOTE: The comparison is expressed as a ratio, with the mean for all hospitals presented as 1.00 and the mean for each sector compared with the grand mean. The difference between the largest and smallest ratio numbers is shown in the last column.
a. American College of Surgeons.
b. Joint Commission on Accreditation of Hospitals.
c. Value of equipment assets per bed in dollars.
d. Average score on facilities and services scale.

Despite the increasing similarity among sectors, it is important to emphasize that each sector exhibits considerable heterogeneity in behavior. Much of the heterogeneity is due to differences in size. The behavior of small hospitals differs greatly from that of large ones, irrespective of ownership. Hospitals of the same size with different types of ownership, however, have become increasingly similar in their behavior.

Irrespective of size, the behavior of hospitals that vary substantially in their sources of funding also differs considerably. This is most apparent in the nation's 100 largest cities, where many voluntary and public hospitals provide substantial care to low-income patients who have little or no third-party coverage. These hospitals often encounter chronic deficits, experience overcrowding, and have fewer full-time-equivalent staff per bed because their sources and levels of funding differ considerably from those of most other short-term hospitals. Their funding problems make them differ greatly from others of comparable size and threaten their ability to provide the same standard of care as other hospitals. As long as hospitals receive funds from different sources or different levels of funding, they will continue to behave differently. Because all hospitals attempt to earn a margin on their revenues, it is questionable how long public or voluntary hospitals can continue to serve large numbers of patients without third-party coverage unless present policies governing funding for large urban hospitals are changed.

Most hospitals encounter much the same problems. Similarly reliant on public revenues, particularly on Medicare, they find themselves squeezed as third-party payers pose new restrictions on reimbursement.

Private and public sources are increasingly pressuring hospitals to narrow the gap between the cost of care and the charges that patients are expected to pay. This difference, which many third-party payers are trying to narrow or eliminate, is the source of most hospital revenue to cover bad debt, charity care, profit, and some of the expenses of teaching and research. Both public regulation and the private marketplace are calling into question the ability of hospitals to maintain their cost reimbursement strategy.

Hospitals in different sectors, as the following chapter discusses, have different options available to them. In their efforts to cope with the reimbursement challenge, they find themselves reexamining their traditional goals, roots, and behavior.

Notes

1. Frank A. Sloan, "Property Rights in the Hospital Industry," in H. E. Frech III, ed., *Health Care in America: Political Economy of Hospitals and Health Insurance* (San Francisco: Pacific Research Institute for Public Policy, forthcoming); and Arnold S. Relman, "Investor-owned Hospitals and Health-Care Costs," *New England Journal of Medicine,* vol. 309 (August 11, 1983) pp. 370–72.

2. J. Rogers Hollingsworth and Ellen Jane Hollingsworth, "Differences between Voluntary and Public Organizations: The Behavior of Hospitals in England and Wales," *Journal of Health Politics, Policy, and Law,* vol. 10 (Summer 1985), pp. 371–97.

3. David D. Rutstein et al., "Measuring the Quality of Medical Care," *New England Journal of Medicine,* vol. 294 (March 11, 1976), pp. 582–88; Milton I. Roemer, A. Taher Moustafa, and Carl F. Hopkins, "A Proposed Hospital Quality Index: Hospital Death Rates Adjusted for Case Severity," *Health Services Research,* vol. 3 (Summer 1968), pp. 113–17; Avedis Donabedian, *Benefits in Medical Care Programs* (Cambridge, Mass.: Harvard University Press, 1976); and Avedis Donabedian, "Promoting Quality through Evaluating the Process of Patient Care," *Medical Care,* vol. 6 (January–February 1968), pp. 181–202. See Appendix for further discussion of quality.

4. Public hospitals in the South were smaller than public hospitals elsewhere, and voluntary hospitals in the Northeast were larger than those elsewhere.

5. Michael M. Davis and C. Rufus Rorem, *The Crisis in Hospital Finance* (Chicago: University of Chicago Press, 1932), p. 149.

6. C. Rufus Rorem, *The Public's Investment in Hospitals* (Chicago: University of Chicago Press, 1930), pp. 171–72, 201; and Haven Emerson, *The Hospitals Survey for New York* (New York: United Hospital Fund, 1937), vol. 1, pp. 217–18.

7. J. H. Hayes, *Financing Hospital Care in the United States* (New York: Blackstone Co., 1954), vol. 1, pp. 52–75; Rorem, *Public's Investment;* Davis and Rorem, *Crisis in Hospital Finance;* and Michael M. Davis, "Who Finances Construction?" *Modern Hospital,* vol. 51 (November 1938), pp. 57–58.

8. Michael M. Davis, "The Indigent Patient and the Voluntary Hospital," *Hospitals,* vol. 13 (July 1939), pp. 32–35; and Emerson, *Hospital Survey,* vol. 1, pp. 23–27.

9. Committee on the Costs of Medical Care, *Medical Care for the American People: The Final Report* (Chicago: University of Chicago Press, 1932), p. 6.

10. Emerson, *Hospital Survey,* vol. 1, pp. 44–46.

11. Davis and Rorem, *Crisis in Hospital Finance,* pp. 141–42; and Emerson, *Hospital Survey,* vol. 1, pp. 32–33, 45–46, 119.

12. *Business Census of Hospitals,* p. 5. See Appendix.

13. Harry Becker, *Financing Hospital Care in the United States* (New York: McGraw Hill Book Company, 1954), vol. 1, p. 11; U.S. Department of Health, Education, and Welfare, Public Health Service, *Medical Care Financing and Utilization* (Washington, D.C., 1962), table 80.

14. Ibid., tables 105, 108.

15. Ibid., table 108.

16. Ibid., table 105.

17. Significant at .05 level.

18. See Appendix for details about construction of index.

19. Committee on Implications of For-Profit Enterprise in Health Care, Institute of Medicine, Bradford H. Gray, ed., *For-Profit Enterprise in Health Care* (Washington, D.C.: National Academy Press, 1986), chap. 5, pp. 97–126. Hereafter cited as Gray, *For-Profit Enterprise*.

20. Edmund R. Becker and Frank A. Sloan, "Hospital Ownership and Performance," *Economic Inquiry*, vol. 23 (January 1985), pp. 21–36; and Carson W. Bays, "Patterns of Hospital Growth," *Medical Care*, vol. 27 (September 1983), pp. 850–57. Hospitals also became more sensitive to the emergence of health maintenance organizations (HMOs) throughout the United States. For an excellent study of how HMOs developed in American cities, see Odin W. Anderson, Terry E. Herold, Bruce W. Butler, Claire H. Kohrman, and Ellen M. Morrison, *HMO Development: Patterns and Prospects* (Chicago: Pluribus Press, 1985).

21. J. Michael Watt, Steven C. Renn, James S. Hahn, Robert A. Derzon, and Carl J. Schramm, "The Effects of Ownership and Multihospital System Membership on Hospital Functional Strategies and Economic Performance," in Gray, *For-Profit Enterprise*, pp. 260–89.

22. Literature discussing hospital efficiency and its relation to size includes R. E. Berry and W. J. Carr, "Efficiency in the Production of Hospital Services" (Report for Social and Rehabilitation Service, Harvard College, June 1973); R. E. Berry, "Product Heterogeneity and Hospital Cost Analysis," *Inquiry*, vol. 7 (March 1970), pp. 67–75; Paul Feldstein, *An Empirical Investigation of the Marginal Cost of Hospital Services* (Chicago: University of Chicago Press, 1961); and Martin Feldstein, *Economic Analysis for Health Service Efficiency* (Amsterdam: North-Holland, 1967).

23. The standard deviation in size in 1979 was 156 for public hospitals and 86 for proprietary hospitals.

24. Becker and Sloan, "Hospital Ownership," p. 25.

25. Ibid. Data since 1979 reveal a comparable trend but with higher percentages of revenue derived from Medicare and Medicaid. This information is made available from Ross Mullner of the American Hospital Association and Frank Sloan of Vanderbilt University. See also Dan Ermann and Jon Gabel, "Multihospital Systems: Issues and Empirical Findings," *Health Affairs*, vol. 3 (Spring 1984), pp. 50–64; and E. Biggs et al., "A Comparison of Contract-managed and Traditionally-managed Non-Profit Hospitals," *Medical Care*, vol. 18 (June 1980), pp. 585–96.

26. Office for Civil Rights, U.S. Department of Health and Human Services. Data reported in Diane Rowland, "Hospital Care for the Uninsured: An Analysis of the Role of Proprietary Hospitals" (Paper presented at the American Public Health Association, Anaheim, California, 1984).

27. Frank A. Sloan, Joseph Valvona, and Ross Mullner, "Identifying the Issues: A Statistical Profile," in Frank A. Sloan, James Blumstein, and James M. Perrin, eds., *Uncompensated Hospital Care: Defining Rights and Assigning*

Responsibilities (Baltimore: Johns Hopkins University Press, 1985), pp. 16–53; Sloan, "Property Rights"; and Gray, *For-Profit Enterprise*, chap. 5, pp. 97–126.

28. Gray, *For-Profit Enterprise*.

29. Florida Hospital Cost Containment Board, *Annual Report, 1983–1984*; Tennessee Department of Health and Environment, unpublished data; Texas Hospital Association, "Survey of Uncompensated Care in Hospitals," *Statement of Fair Share Formula for Financing Care for the Medically Indigent* (Texas Hospital Association, 1985); Virginia Health Services Cost Review Commission, unpublished data; and Gray, *For-Profit Enterprise*.

30. See Judith Feder, Jack Hadley, and Ross Mullner, "Falling through the Cracks: Poverty, Insurance Coverage, and Hospital Care for the Poor, 1980 and 1982," *Health and Society*, vol. 62 (1984), pp. 544–66; Sloan, Valvona, and Mullner, "Identifying the Issues"; and Robert V. Pattison and Hallie M. Katz, "Investor-owned and Not-for-Profit Hospitals," *New England Journal of Medicine*, vol. 309 (August 11, 1983), pp. 347–53.

31. Feder, Hadley, and Mullner, "Falling through the Cracks"; Robert Wood Johnson Foundation, *An Updated Report on Access to Health Care for the American People* (Princeton, N.J.: Robert Wood Johnson Foundation, 1983); and Gray, *For-Profit Enterprise*.

32. See the interesting paper by Deborah Freund, Richard H. Shachtman, Marshall Ruffin, and Dana Quade, "Analysis of Length-of-Stay Differences between Investor-owned and Voluntary Hospitals," *Inquiry*, vol. 22 (Spring 1985), pp. 33–44. See also Charles A. Register, Ansel M. Sharp, and David G. Bivin, "Profit Incentives and the Hospital Industry: Are We Expecting Too Much?" *Health Services Research*, vol. 20 (June 1985), pp. 225–41. For state studies demonstrating that case mix varied by ownership, see Carson W. Bays, "Case-Mix Differences between Non-Profit and For-Profit Hospitals," *Inquiry*, vol. 14 (March 1977), pp. 19–23; and Carson W. Bays, "Cost Comparisons of For-Profit and Non-Profit Hospitals," *Social Science Medicine*, vol. 13 (1979), pp. 219–55. For a discussion of the relation between length of stay and case mix, see Judith Lave and S. Leinhart, "The Cost and Length of a Hospital Stay," *Inquiry*, vol. 13 (1976), pp. 327–43.

33. See. H. S. Ruchlin, D. D. Point, and L. L. Cannedy, "A Comparison of For-Profit and Investor-owned Chain and Nonprofit Hospitals," *Inquiry*, vol. 10 (1973), pp. 13–23; and Register et al., "Profit Incentives." For a finding that for-profit hospitals in California, Texas, and Florida used fewer full-time-equivalent employees per occupied bed than voluntary hospitals, see Lawrence S. Lewin et al., "Investor Owneds and Nonprofits Differ in Economic Performances," *Hospitals*, vol. 55 (July 1981), pp. 52–58. See also Joseph S. Coyne, "Health Performance in Multihospital Systems: A Comparative Study of System and Independent Hospitals," *Health Services Research*, vol. 17 (Winter 1982), pp. 303–29.

34. Presentation of Michael D. Bromberg to Institute of Medicine Committee, March 15, 1984; Michael A. Morrisey, Jeffrey A. Alexander, and Stephen M. Shortell, "Medical Staff Size, Hospital Privileges, and Compensation Arrangements: A Comparison of System Hospitals," in Gray, *For-Profit Enterprise*, pp. 422–57; and Robert A. Musacchio et al., "Hospital Ownership and

the Practice of Medicine: Evidence from the Physician's Perspective," in Gray, *For-Profit Enterprise.*

35. Morrisey et al., "Medical Staff Size."

36. Ibid.; and Musacchio et al., "Hospital Ownership."

37. Musacchio et al., "Hospital Ownership."

38. Jeffrey A. Alexander, Michael A. Morrisey, and Stephen M. Shortell, "Physician Participation in the Administration and Governance of System and Freestanding Hospitals: A Comparison by Type of Ownership," in Gray, *For-Profit Enterprise,* pp. 402–21; and Musacchio et al., "Hospital Ownership."

39. Daniel R. Longo et al., "Compliance of Multi-hospital Systems with JCAH Standards" (Report for the Institute of Medicine Committee on Implications of For-Profit Enterprise in Health Care, 1985).

40. Frank A. Sloan and Robert A. Vraciu, "Investor-owned and Not-for-Profit Hospitals: Addressing Some Issues," *Health Affairs,* vol. 2 (Spring 1983), pp. 34–35.

41. Watt et al., "Effects of Ownership"; Craig G. Coelen, "Hospital Ownership and Comparative Hospital Costs," in Gray, *For-Profit Enterprise,* pp. 322–53; and Becker and Sloan, "Hospital Ownership." Coelen excludes public hospitals.

42. Becker and Sloan, "Hospital Ownership."

43. Robert V. Pattison, "Response to Financial Incentives among Investor-Owned and Not-for-Profit Hospitals: An Analysis Based on California Data, 1978–1982," in Gray, *For-Profit Enterprise,* pp. 290–302; and Kathryn J. Brown and Richard E. Klosterman, "Hospital Acquisitions and Their Effects: Florida, 1979–1982," in Gray, *For-Profit Enterprise,* pp. 303–21.

44. Regina E. Herzlinger and William S. Krasker, "Who Profits from Non-profits?" *Harvard Business Review,* vol. 65 (January–February 1987), pp. 93–106. See also Letters to the Editor, *Harvard Business Review,* vol. 65 (March–April 1987), pp. 134–52.

45. Sloan and Vraciu, "Investor-owned Hospitals."

46. Lewin et al., "Investor Owneds"; Pattison and Katz, "Investor-owned Hospitals"; J. Michael Watt et al., "The Comparative Economic Performance of Investor-owned Chain and Not-for-Profit Hospitals," *New England Journal of Medicine,* vol. 314 (January 9, 1986), pp. 89–96; and Pattison, "Response to Financial Incentives."

47. Sloan and Vraciu, "Investor-owned Hospitals"; Phyllis Taylor, Louis D. Leary, and William J. Bennet, "The Continuing Dialogue on Expenses in Investor-owned Hospitals" (Report for the Institute of Medicine Committee on Implications of For-Profit Enterprise in Health Care, 1985); Sloan, "Property Rights"; and Robin Eskoz and Michael Peddecord, "The Relationship of Hospital Ownership and Service Composition to Hospital Charges," *Health Care Financing Review,* vol. 6 (Spring 1985), pp. 51–58. For an earlier study, see B. Ferber, "An Analysis of Chain-operated For-Profit Hospitals," *Health Services Research,* vol. 6 (Spring 1971), pp. 49–60.

48. Gray, *For-Profit Enterprise.*

49. Becker and Sloan, "Hospital Ownership"; Watt et al., "Comparative Performance"; and Coelen, "Hospital Ownership."

50. Gray, *For-Profit Enterprise*.

51. Becker and Sloan, "Hospital Ownership"; Sloan and Vraciu, "Investor-owned Hospitals"; Lewin et al., "Investor Owneds"; and Pattison and Katz, "Investor-owned Hospitals."

52. Margaret B. Sulvetta, "Public Hospital Provision of Care to the Poor and Financial Status," Working Paper, Urban Institute, Washington, D.C., 1985; Jack Hadley and Judith Feder, "Hospitals' Financial Status and Care to the Poor," Working Paper, Urban Institute, Washington, D.C., 1983, Executive Summary.

53. Data for 1983 provided by Frank Sloan, from American Hospital Association annual survey.

4
Responses to a Changing Environment

This chapter is concerned with how the three hospital sectors are likely to adjust to problems confronting the American hospital industry during the next decade. It focuses on three problems: pressures to limit hospitals' operating budgets; the need for new capital; and the provision of uncompensated care. Of course, a myriad of other problems confront American hospitals, though less urgently. These three problems are interrelated and overlap, even though we make some effort to treat them separately. Each problem is briefly described, and the likely responses of each sector are discussed. The sectors vary somewhat in the extent to which they are affected by the problems and in their ability to cope with them. The for-profit sector has exerted influence on each of these problems in recent years both as a model for behavior and as a competitive force.[1]

Pressures to Limit Hospitals' Operating Budgets

The explanation for the budgetary problems facing many American hospitals is familiar—declines in rates of occupancy, changes in medical technology, changes in methods of reimbursing hospitals, increased competition among hospitals and between physicians and hospitals, and greater ability of third-party payers to bargain about rates. Since 1980 hospital occupancy rates have fallen, admissions for those under age sixty-five have declined, and average stays in hospitals have become shorter. In a single year—from 1983 to 1984—hospitals experienced a decline of 7.8 percent in total patient days.[2] About 40 percent of hospital beds were empty in 1986, and Joseph Califano, former secretary of health, education, and welfare, has talked of eliminating 400,000–500,000 beds nationwide.[3] At the same time many hospitals have employed more staff as they have added more complex equipment. And costs have continued to rise, although their rate of growth has decreased. For many hospitals funds have not increased proportionately.[4] The noted economist Uwe Reinhardt has suggested that the fall in costs is illusory and that costs are continuing to grow at an alarming rate.[5]

Demographic and economic changes have also affected hospitals. Flight away from central cities has often left older, downtown hospitals without sufficient paying clients. Hospitals in many cities have excess capacity, forcing them to compete for clients. Estimates are that New York, Chicago, and a few other large cities have a bed surplus of 25 percent.[6] The New York City Health Systems Agency has called for a 14 percent cut in public hospital beds and even for the municipal government to get out of the hospital business.[7]

Another source of pressure on operating budgets has been the ability of third-party payers to bargain with hospitals about rates. Although in some states Medicaid authorities and Blue Cross have for many years bargained about rates or secured discounts, such practices are now becoming widespread among health maintenance organizations (HMOs) and self-insuring groups. Nationally HMOs have approximately 17 million members, and membership is increasing about 20 percent annually.

Meanwhile, the number of hospital admissions has declined somewhat because of increased cost sharing by patients. A number of large employers are incorporating higher deductible or coinsurance amounts in their employee health benefit plans. One recent study of 1,200 companies found that slightly more than 50 percent included deductibles in their employee plans in 1984, in contrast to only 17 percent two years earlier. Moreover, many insurance plans now require preadmission authorization, second opinions for elective surgery, or postdischarge planning.[8]

Technological innovations are changing the site for the delivery of many medical services. Many services formerly provided to inpatients are now offered outside the hospital, and new technologies have reduced recovery periods and lengths of stay. Moreover, free-standing emergency centers and surgicenters are competing with hospitals for patients.

Of course, the major actor affecting hospital reimbursement has been the federal government, as it has implemented a system of diagnosis-related groups (DRGs) for Medicare patients. For many years the federal government reimbursed hospitals for inpatient services under the Medicare program on the basis of "reasonable and necessary" costs. This reimbursement system gave hospitals and doctors incentives to overtreat patients. The DRG system of paying a fixed amount based on a specific diagnosis has radically changed reimbursement. Now hospitals have incentives to decrease the length of stay of elderly patients, to reduce the number and cost of ancillary services, and to substitute low-cost for high-cost technologies.

States have also made serious efforts to limit hospital costs. As state regulation has become more stringent, more and more hospitals have been subject to rate and budget review, with financial penalties for performance shortfalls. Restrictive payment practices for Medicaid by both states and the federal government and constraints on care for the poor have led to less use of hospitals by low-income groups and less hospital income.

These combined pressures seem overpowering for some hospitals that only a few years ago were able to secure financial resources and administer care without great difficulty. Yet the financial status of American hospitals is mixed. A substantial minority of hospitals, especially large urban public hospitals, are in chronic financial trouble. Stressed hospitals in large urban areas (either public or voluntary) are three times as likely as stressed rural hospitals to have experienced a deficit in each of the past three years.[9]

Despite the pressure on operating budgets, various signs—apart from improved profit margins—suggest that financial conditions are not dire for most hospitals. Favorable margins for most hospitals suggest that stress on operating margins has been manageable. Net revenue margins for all community hospitals increased from 0.7 percent in 1975 to 3.6 percent in 1981 and to 6.2 percent in 1984.[10] Earnings were 6.7 percent of revenue for the first eight months of 1985 and 5.2 percent for 1986.[11]

Although the federal government has claimed an annual reduction of $2 billion in Medicare hospital payments due to DRGs, there is strong evidence that hospitals are showing profits of 12–18 percent on Medicare patients. An 18 percent profit would mean that for every dollar a hospital received from Medicare, it would spend eighty-two cents for patient care.[12] Even so, hospitals have battled furiously for greater percentage increases in DRG reimbursement than the Reagan administration has been willing to provide.

Although hospital closures have been widely forecast, only 156 hospitals closed between 1980 and 1984, a very small number compared with the thousands continuing to provide care. In fact, a smaller proportion of hospitals closed in recent years—whether during the past five or the past ten years—than in a comparable period before the introduction of Medicare and Medicaid. Of those that closed between 1980 and 1984 approximately 80 percent had fewer than 100 beds, and about 70 percent were either in small communities unable to support hospitals or in cities with more than 2.5 million people, where they succumbed to intense competition.[13] Both closings and low occupancy are signs of oversupply—a situation familiar in other sectors but uncharacteristic of American hospitals.

Most hospitals have resorted to a variety of tactics to cope with

127

resource scarcity, although responses to the rapidly changing environments vary among the three kinds of hospitals. Yet individual hospitals are experiencing considerable uncertainty about their future. Many of the oldest and most prestigious hospitals in the nation are far more uncertain about their future than they were sixty years ago.[14]

The Voluntary Sector. Hospitals in the voluntary sector have undertaken a number of actions to cope with their environmental uncertainty. In many large cities some rationalization of specialized services among voluntary hospitals is taking place to reduce duplication. In some communities area planning is becoming common.

Probably the most significant activity has been greater participation of voluntary hospitals in multi-institutional organizations. Frank Sloan estimates the rate of growth among private nonprofit chains at 11.4 percent per year from 1978 to 1982. Although other scholars have different estimates, it is obvious that multi-institutional arrangements are becoming more common among private nonprofit hospitals.[15] From 1983 to 1984 the "profits" or surplus of nonreligious hospitals in nonprofit chains increased faster than the profits of investor-owned chains.[16] Their variety is substantial, as indicated in chapter 2. Some arrangements are across sectoral lines, especially as nonprofit voluntary hospitals seek management by other hospitals or by for-profit organizations.

Vertical integration is proliferating in the voluntary sector as hospitals scramble to increase their margins or to avoid losses. Some are expanding into new markets—into the provision of home care services, nursing home care, alcoholism and mental health treatment services, medical insurance, and HMOs. Some are constructing office space for doctors in adjacent buildings and are providing subsidized rents to attract doctors and patients. Many large organizations are no longer in one of the three sectors but are hybrids. Some for-profit organizations have nonprofit research units, and numerous nonprofit hospitals are involved in for-profit real estate ventures.[17]

Not all voluntary hospital changes are adaptations to the environment; many changes are taking place within the hospital. Some hospitals have improved their financial management and accounting services, through use of both electronic equipment and trained analysts, especially as the communications revolution has made storage and analysis of data more routine. Many have eliminated services and staffs that lose money and have avoided the introduction of new services, such as trauma and burn centers, that are not self-financing. New services are not routinely avoided, however, for some kinds of new units are being created, especially if they earn profits. Special injury care units try to attract automobile accident victims, who usually carry hospital insurance.[18]

Aggressive marketing to both individuals and groups has become much more extensive. In some communities media advertising has become intense as hospitals attempt to keep occupancy rates high to meet fixed costs. Billboards on highways and on top of buildings have become common means of advertising the medical facilities of both individual hospitals and their chain affiliates. As hospitals expand their outpatient services, some have resorted to providing overnight convenience care in association with those services. Many voluntary hospitals are reducing uncompensated care through the reduction of charitable care and more selective admissions of self-paying patients. In many locations the transfer of low or no-pay patients to public hospitals has increased. Throughout the country voluntary hospitals are attempting to model themselves after for-profit hospitals.[19]

Obviously, the extent to which these measures are being undertaken varies, and their efficacy in reducing budget pressures is mixed. For the large voluntary hospitals in the center of the nation's biggest cities—those with heavy charity caseloads—such actions are not likely to be able to stem fiscal pressures. They cannot recruit new charge-paying patients, and reductions in cost-paying patients may mean empty beds and less affordable overhead. Small free-standing hospitals are similarly troubled.

The Public Sector. Changes among public hospitals are also geared to adapting the hospital to changes in its environment and to management changes. Public hospitals are also participating in some rationalization of services, both within the public sector and across sectoral lines. Reorganization is occurring as some public hospitals join with voluntary and for-profit organizations in hybrid networks permitting economies of scale. Some public hospitals are becoming parts of other public organizations.[20] Some are hiring for-profit firms to provide emergency room services or turning over their entire administration to proprietary organizations.[21]

Many public hospitals are dramatically improving their financial and other management and are more vigorously pursuing third-party and self-pay reimbursement. Hospitals substantially dependent on local public funding agencies are becoming increasingly aggressive in their presentations to such agencies.

It is difficult to appraise how well these measures will succeed in relieving the pressures on operating budgets. The public hospital sector is very heterogeneous (as well as very large), and generalizations about some public hospitals are inapplicable to others. Regardless of these measures, major public hospitals in large cities will continue to face daunting budget pressures, an experience with which they are entirely familiar. Whatever their efforts to enhance accountability to patients and to maintain high-quality care, they recognize that they have a very special status. As facilities of last resort in areas inhabited by the poor, most cannot easily be closed. They may be denied opportunities for upgrading their standards, but their survival is not usually in doubt, although they are being forced to cut back on services and in some the quality of care is being threatened.

The debate over New York City's hospitals exemplifies a lack of consensus about larger public hospitals. The hospitals are accused of a shortage of professional staff and equipment,[22] even asked to turn their functions over to voluntary hospitals.[23] Some observers, however, compliment the hospitals of the city, public as well as voluntary, for their lean operations but recognize that new investment in capital equipment is necessary.[24]

Quite aware that a sizable budget share comes from public authorities, the administrators of large public hospitals spend considerable time cultivating elected and appointed public officials, making a convincing case that their services are indispensable in a society with any vestige of social conscience. With somewhat lower costs per day and per stay, public hospitals can avoid most allegations of waste and inefficiency. However persuasive their cases and however effective their management, many financially stressed public hospitals are presenting their arguments to public authorities at a time when the entire public sector is in financial difficulties. The fiscal problems of the large public hospital mirror the fiscal problems of the city or county government, which usually has few resources to spare.[25]

Although the burden of appropriating substantial sums for hospital budgets may be onerous for many public authorities, the prospect of selling a hospital or letting it remove itself from public authority is unacceptable to most communities. Most public hospitals have limited potential to become part of chains or to enter into system arrangements. In some states public authorities have threatened to prohibit the conveyance of public hospitals to for-profit auspices.[26] Public hospitals are likely, however, to become increasingly involved in arrangements with voluntary or for-profit organizations, since such hybrid arrangements offer chances to rationalize services, achieve economies of scale, and mitigate social responsibility.

The For-Profit Sector. Although the analytical literature is mixed in its findings and the evidence is not clear, investor-owned hospitals will most likely experience very little financial stress in the near future, although they might experience a decline in profits. Before 1983 their costs to patients were higher than those of other hospitals of comparable size (see chapter 3), but it is fairly clear that their margins were also higher than those of hospitals in either the voluntary or the public sector. These profit margins may not have been what investor-owned chains desired, of course, and how high they are in the DRG era remains somewhat uncertain.

Because most for-profit hospitals are located in states without severe regulatory climates, they are more likely, in the short term, to avoid some of the more stringent pressures to reduce operating revenues. Four states (New Jersey, Maryland, New York, and Massachusetts) now have all-payer regulatory rate schemes, and it is not accidental that the number of proprietary hospitals in these states is very small. Because for-profit hospitals are located in areas experiencing population growth, they may be able to maintain adequate occupancy rates and keep profit margins high even if national trends for voluntary and public hospitals move in the opposite direction.

Those for-profit hospitals that experience financial stress will not be subject to the strong pressures of local public authorities or local boards of trustees. With 80 percent of for-profit hospitals in large chains, most decisions about how to confront stress on budgets will not be taken locally, although this will vary from one chain to another. For-profit hospitals can close beds, close units, or close entirely without much public scrutiny. With occupancy down to 45 percent in 1985—compared with 63 percent industry-wide—some investor-owned hospitals are now at risk.[27]

Well accustomed to managing by budget and financial information, for-profit hospitals will continue to seek innovative means of spreading overhead (through management contracts, for example) and of controlling staff costs. Always attentive to the volume of uncompensated care and not traditionally associated with charitable care in any large amount, for-profit hospitals will be far more sensitive than public or voluntary hospitals to decisions that require shifting of costs. And if DRGs or other changes in reimbursement reduce the profit margins of proprietary chains, they have considerable flexibility to sell off unprofitable operations and to move into profitable activities—not only in areas related to health, such as HMOs, home care services, and health insurance, but also into sectors of the economy completely unrelated to health care.

For-profit hospitals are increasingly linked in very large and diversified health care organizations. Humana, for example, has become very active in offering HMOs, and the Hospital Corporation of

America (HCA) is now following suit.[28] As parts of large international vertically and horizontally integrated organizations, many for-profit hospitals will be able to overcome temporary budgetary pressures. The factors long associated with the for-profit sector—flexibility and speed in responding to changes in the marketplace—should serve it well in avoiding and controlling financial stress.

Yet investor-owned chains are experiencing some difficulties. In early 1987 it was reported that they were dumping costly acute-care hospitals and retreating from their forays into insurance and HMOs.[29]

Raising Capital for Hospitals

There is widespread agreement that the need for capital in the hospital industry will be considerable in the coming decade. The estimated needs vary widely, however—from $100 billion to $200 billion.[30] Whatever estimate is correct, the need for capital poses complex public policy issues. Raising capital is a common problem, of course, in all sectors of the economy. The means available to hospitals have become more like those used in other industries.

How is the capital to be raised, and how is society to determine how much capital is actually needed? Many observers argue that the United States invests too much capital in the hospital industry. One difficulty is that we do not know how to measure needs, especially in sectors of the economy of great technological complexity where the technology changes very rapidly. One way of assessing need is to examine the age of the hospital, which can influence replacement timing and cost. For accounting purposes the useful life of hospital plants has been estimated at twenty-five years.[31] Focusing on both plant and equipment, a 1980 study by ICF concluded that about 93 percent of community hospital assets were less than fifteen years old and 76 percent were less than ten years old. Unfortunately, no reliable published data disaggregate the age of plant and equipment.[32]

We know that future capital needs vary greatly from one part of the country to another. Some areas will need capital sooner than others. Many hospitals were built between 1948 and 1970 with Hill-Burton funding, when fuel was plentiful and inexpensive. Although many are not very old, a sizable proportion of them are not energy efficient, many are poorly designed to house new kinds of technology, and many need renovation. In New Jersey, Massachusetts, and New York, many older buildings require costly renovation, structural redesign, or outright replacement. A sizable proportion of hospitals in the South, Southwest, and Far West are much younger and have more moderate capital needs.

132

A cross-national perspective permits a somewhat different assessment. The hospital stock in Britain is much older than in the United States; yet there is virtually no evidence that the quality of patient care has suffered. For many years the British government quite consciously skimped on capital for hospitals. The British case makes the point that the needs for hospital capital cannot be precisely and objectively defined, that the problem clearly has a cultural dimension. British professionals are obviously willing to accept hospital plants and equipment that would be unacceptable to Americans. Many U.S. physicians are unwilling to work in a hospital unless it has the latest facilities. Thus measuring the need for capital by ascertaining the investment in hospitals in other countries at a comparable level of development is limited. The amount of capital to be invested in American hospitals is in many respects a political question.[33]

How have decisions about the source of capital been made in the past? What role has the state played? What proposals are currently being made to cope with the problem of capital? How is capital for the hospital industry likely to be generated in the future?

Before the Second World War the primary sources of capital for hospitals were philanthropy and patients' fees. In 1946 the federal government began to be a major source of capital for voluntary and public hospitals. Moreover, the emergence of widespread private health insurance did much to improve hospitals' access to debt financing. The insurance industry established the precedent of third-party payers' funding depreciation, interest, and reserves for capital expenditure, and this precedent was later incorporated in Medicare and Medicaid policies. Moreover, the establishment of mortgage loan and insurance programs for voluntary and investor-owned hospitals under Section 242 of the Federal Housing Act dramatically improved hospitals' access to debt financing for capital expenditures. It was the emergence of tax-exempt revenue bonds between 1971 and 1977, however, that enabled many hospitals to engage in debt financing. During these years tax-exempt financing increased at an annual rate of 52 percent, adjusted for inflation.[34]

Under Medicare much debt was indirectly financed by the federal government, which reimbursed the Medicare portion of hospital capital costs due to interest and depreciation. In addition, it paid proprietary hospitals a return on equity capital. Even after 1983, when Medicare abandoned cost-based reimbursement in favor of a prospective payment system, hospitals were still reimbursed directly for capital costs.

It is important to recognize that government regulatory accounting techniques are not neutral but are instruments that serve economic interests. This has clearly been true of Medicare. Receiving

133

much of their capital revenue from cost-based reimbursement, hospitals have had a strong incentive to maximize reimbursement rather than to minimize capital investment. Their behavior has responded to government incentives. Since the federal government and commercial insurers reimbursed hospitals for much of their depreciation and interest, hospitals became increasingly active in raising capital through debt.

The growth of multihospital chains was also related to debt financing. First, in seeking debt capital, hospitals had an incentive to pool their revenues to gain more favorable access to the credit markets and lower interest rates. Chain arrangements were attractive because they provided a larger base of operations over which to spread costs. Second, with the federal government paying a large portion of interest and depreciation, there were incentives to increase holdings by borrowing. If newly acquired hospitals were expensive—and mergers generally cost a great deal—they were less difficult to manage by the acquiring hospital if the federal government was helping to pay for them.

The investor-owned segment of the hospital industry has been especially aggressive in taking advantage of this strategy. The resultant mergers substantially increased federal outlays for capital expenditures, as the 1981 merger between the HCA and Hospital Affiliates International (HAI) shows. A General Accounting Office study demonstrated that the merger increased hospital depreciation, interest, and home office costs by $55 million in the first year after the acquisition. Much of the increase was attributable, however, to depreciation expenses resulting from asset revaluation. Furthermore, asset revaluation increased the equity basis on which return on equity was calculated. The total capital costs due to the consolidation increased 28 percent in the year following merger.[35]

Medicare methods of reimbursement for capital costs have been the same for voluntary and for-profit hospitals, with one exception: voluntary hospitals do not receive a return on equity. The incentive structure for capital reimbursement was the same for both—to maximize capital investments. Thus Medicare has made large capital payments to hospitals that have been credit worthy, have had good access to capital markets, and have invested heavily in capital equipment. Conversely, Medicare has made smaller capital payments to hospitals not active in capital markets—large urban public hospitals and hospitals in small towns.

How to reimburse hospitals for capital expenditures under Medicare is much discussed. The two proposals that have received the most attention are (1) a continuation of the cost-based reimbursement program, which encourages capital investment, and (2) a plan, supported by the Reagan administration, that incorporates payment for capital into the DRG program of prospective reimbursement.

Under the first plan Medicare capital would continue to flow to hospitals most active in the credit markets, very likely those with the greatest surpluses. Hospitals in chronic financial stress, less able to attract capital, would receive less Medicare reimbursement to improve their capital stock.

Under the second plan, with capital incorporated into the DRG-based payments, capital reimbursement would be linked to Medicare volume and to case mix rather than to total fixed costs. Hospitals serving large numbers of Medicare patients and having higher-cost case mixes would receive more Medicare payments than those with smaller Medicare volumes and lower-cost case mixes. Capital costs would be factored in prospectively rather than paid retrospectively. The incorporation of prospective payment for capital into the DRG payment would do much to reduce incentives to spend unnecessary capital in hospitals. The total capital reimbursement from Medicare would be reduced, and dollars for capital would "follow the patient." Although much of the recent discussion has focused on the second plan, it does not solve all the problems of raising capital for the nation's hospitals, for Medicare alone cannot provide for all the future needs of hospitals.

The overwhelming majority of hospital capital is now raised through debt. Hospitals that fare best in the capital markets are part of multihospital arrangements and have high-quality management, a low percentage of uncompensated care, a favorable debt capacity, and higher operating margins. During a twenty-one-month period of 1979–1980, 72 percent of multihospitals' bond issues and only 17 percent of unaffiliated hospitals' bond issues received an AA rating or higher. If this trend were to continue unabated, investor-owned and voluntary hospitals in multi-institutional arrangements would probably continue to be successful in raising capital, but free-standing, unaffiliated hospitals would find it difficult—especially hospitals in small towns and those in large urban areas where many patients receive free care.[36]

The outlook is not bright for public hospitals in large urban areas or in small towns to meet their capital needs over the next decade. For smaller voluntary hospitals, access to capital may be greatly enhanced by association with major or flagship hospitals. The need for capital will undoubtedly encourage more voluntary hospitals to enter multi-institutional arrangements.[37]

If some hospitals encountered severe problems in obtaining capital for a prolonged period, serious inequities in care would eventually result. A number of hospitals might have to close because of their location or their combination of payers even though their services were much needed. To avoid such a trend, the federal government may well find that something resembling a Hill-Burton program will be necessary for hospitals unable to obtain adequate capital. Instead of using the capital markets, hospitals designated as serving low-income patients and in desperate need of capital might receive capital subsidies directly from the federal government. The alternative for many free-standing hospitals is likely to be increased financial hardship, reduced services, and deterioration of plant.

Capital needs and plans for voluntary hospitals are likely to be examined much more closely than in the recent past, even with certificate-of-need controls. Rationalization and specialization of services, carried out in the interests of greater efficiency, may give certain kinds of capital spending priority over others. If voluntary hospitals believe that they can do better in occupancy and reimbursement by providing certain kinds of specialized services, those services will have first call on capital. One implication is that voluntary hospitals will be even less likely to provide community-oriented facilities that are not self-supporting or profitable.

Capital needs are likely to be somewhat less intense among for-profit hospitals in the coming decade than in the past decade and also less intense than in the public and voluntary sectors. The major investor-owned chains are no longer buying or building hospitals at the same rate, partly because of a perception that earning profits on hospitals has become more difficult. Moreover, extensive capital investment has already been carried out in recent years in most proprietary hospitals. They are somewhat newer than hospitals in the two other sectors, and their need for capital should be lower. If they establish more free-standing centers with specialized services, however, they may well require substantial additional capital.

Uncompensated Care

Approximately 35 million people in the United States had no hospital insurance and were not covered by Medicaid in 1984. Califano suggested in early 1987 that 37 million would be a more current figure; other experts estimate 39.7 million—about one-sixth of the U.S. population.[38] The number of people without such protection has increased greatly in the past decade, and the question of how they will be cared for when they need hospitalization is critical. In one recent year 9 percent of the U.S. population had no medical insurance, and another

136

8 percent were without insurance during part of the year. Moreover, the uninsured had substantially lower rates of hospital use: forty-seven patient days per 100 population for the uninsured versus ninety per 100 population for the insured.[39] Estimates are that 50 million people have inadequate medical insurance, as throughout the 1980s the percentage of the indigent covered by Medicaid has fallen considerably. Indeed, by early 1987 only 38 percent of the indigent were covered.[40]

Given the enormous number of people without hospital insurance, it is no surprise that the volume of uncompensated care in hospitals has risen steeply. And of course "uncompensated care," a hospital accounting term, does nothing to reflect care unsought or denied because of poverty. The uncompensated care figures for recent years are 1980, $3.5 billion; 1984, $5.7 billion; 1985, $7.4 billion; and 1986, $8 billion.[41] These are indeed very large amounts of money. For example, the $7.4 billion figure for 1985 was 4.6 percent of all hospital revenue.

The potential crisis results from changes in the reimbursement of hospital care affecting the structural arrangements that had paid for the hospital needs of many poor Americans. In the past hospitals have paid for the care of those unable to cover their own expenses in various ways. Most uncompensated care (both charity care and bad debt) has been provided by public hospitals in major metropolitan areas, philanthropic donations, and cost shifting, that is, charging some patients more than others because some do not pay an appropriate share of the costs incurred. These arrangements are rapidly becoming inadequate to deal with the very large number of people without third-party coverage. Large public hospitals in the nation's largest cities are increasingly finding it difficult to serve all the patients turning to them for care; neither their facilities nor their budgets are capable of so much expansion. Philanthropy cannot pay more than a small portion of the bills for uncompensated care. And cost shifting is slowly being abandoned, however involuntarily.[42]

Scholars do not agree about cost shifting. We do not know how extensive it has been, how much money has been involved, how long it has taken place in each sector, or how well it has performed. Some data indicate that the difference between hospital costs and charges was relatively stable during the late 1960s (5 to 7 percent), but by 1979 it was approximately 15 percent. This, of course, is a crude indicator of cost shifting, since some patients paid neither costs nor charges, but the data demonstrate that an increasing percentage of costs had shifted to those willing to pay higher bills.[43]

Many third-party payers that once paid charges (that is, more than actual costs) are changing their policies. Led by the Health Insurance Association of America, many commercial insurance companies, which traditionally reimbursed hospitals at more generous rates, are no longer willing to do so. Many large employers have begun to self-insure and are thereby escaping the burdens of financing uncompensated care through cost shifts. Meanwhile, Blue Cross plans have become more conscious about bargaining for rates, in an effort to contain costs. According to one source, Blue Cross pays only 87 percent of hospital bills. HMOs, also bargaining for hospital rates, are unwilling to bear shifted costs. Medicare has always refused to pay any portion of bad debts or charity not directly attributed to its beneficiaries. According to the Health Insurance Association of America, the difference between what Medicare and Medicaid pay and what private sector patients pay increased from $1.1 billion in 1975 to $3 billion in 1979, $4.8 billion in 1981, and $5.8 billion in 1982.[44] And so it goes, with payer after payer refusing to pay more than costs. Hospitals, confronted with efforts to reduce the cost-shifting cushion, struggling to cope with the financial effects of DRGs, and underpaid by Medicaid, no longer have a convenient way to handle the demands for uncompensated care.

The attack on cost shifting also has implications for medical education and research. Since relatively few hospitals are heavily involved in education and research, however, the issue of funding education and research has drawn less attention than the funding of uncompensated care.[45]

The Voluntary Sector. In 1982 voluntary hospitals provided 60.3 percent of the nation's uncompensated care—from 3.7 percent of all voluntary hospital charges in metropolitan areas to 4 percent in nonmetropolitan areas. The hospitals obviously vary in the extent to which they have suffered serious financial difficulties by providing such care. In general, the demands for uncompensated care are greater in hospitals with strong teaching commitments, metropolitan locations, and sizable Medicaid caseloads. Large eastern teaching hospitals, providing a higher percentage of charitable care than other hospitals, have experienced the most financial stress. Not all teaching hospitals have the same problems, however; some are well situated financially, with doctors of high prestige and abundant charge-paying clients.[46] Many religious hospitals, especially those with a Catholic affiliation, have made extra efforts to shoulder the burden of uncompensated care, keeping alive the ethical principles underlying their foundation.

The possibility of a return by voluntary hospitals to the roots of

138

the voluntary tradition as a means of financing uncompensated care is much discussed. Richard Foster and Robert Sigmond have, in rather different approaches, pointed out that the voluntary hospitals once had an almost unique role as one of the most important institutions in the community serving the poor. By proclaiming and carrying out more community functions, by making it explicit that the care of the poor is something they expect to do, voluntary hospitals might revive some of their former sources of income and raise funds locally to carry greater burdens of charity care. This strategy would obviously call for more of the responsibility for financing uncompensated care to fall directly on the voluntary hospital, which would have to demonstrate that charity care is needed, that the hospital can and will provide it, and that the community should share the costs.[47]

Certainly, the work of Rosemary Stevens has pointed out that at one time many voluntary hospitals received financial assistance from state or local authorities. If voluntary hospitals, Sigmond argues, were delivering significant amounts of charitable care, they could convince the public of their community service mission and thus once again address the goals for which they were initially intended. If they do not revive their tradition of serving the indigent, they will increasingly risk losing their nonprofit status, especially if their behavior continues to resemble that of investor-owned hospitals.[48]

There are problems with returning to community roots, however. It has been suggested that the hospital often arose more from segmented interest groups than from the whole community. Many voluntary hospitals had their origins not in donations and philanthropy but in services for fees. Since the Second World War many hospitals have become increasingly sensitive to the medical-industrial complex and less concerned with local responsibilities. For all these reasons, going back to the community may not be easy.[49]

Instead of increasing their responsibility for the poor, voluntary hospitals will probably make greater efforts to minimize their responsibility and to reduce the costs of uncompensated care. They are likely to reduce costs by refusing admission to those unable to pay, by eliminating departments or services in which there are high proportions of bad debts (such as self-paying clients in maternity wards), by earlier discharges, by increasing transfers to public institutions, and by reducing ancillary services for nonpaying clients. The stories about patient dumping have drawn so much attention that Congress has enacted penalties for transfer of Medicare patients in unstable condition.[50]

The hospitals may also pursue another alternative. They may use their influence to have the state reduce the amount of uncompensated care. Specifically, they may work for state reimbursement arrangements under which they have access to public funds for disproportionate charitable care. All-payer plans are one strategy that spreads the burden of uncompensated care more equitably among all users of hospitals.[51] Special extra DRG allowances have been created for hospitals providing disproportionate shares of uncompensated care.[52]

Finally, in an effort to obtain funds for uncompensated care, voluntary hospitals might become more involved in hybrid arrangements and attempt to generate a surplus through for-profit enterprises. Although hybrid arrangements are becoming more common among voluntary hospitals, there is very little evidence that they are being entered into to finance uncompensated care.

The Public Sector. In thinking about uncompensated care by public hospitals, it is necessary once again to make some distinctions among the major kinds of public hospitals, as set forth in chapter 2. The problems of uncompensated care vary greatly among public hospitals.

We turn first to the big public hospitals in the nation's largest cities. They have traditionally provided a very disproportionate amount of charitable care, covering most of the costs through public appropriation. Many of them have had limited experience with charge-paying patients. In fact, some have been prohibited from serving such patients; even when they could legally accept charge-paying patients, many have made little effort to attract them. The demise of cost shifting does not occasion much distress among these hospitals.

The load of uncompensated care for these hospitals is very heavy, however, especially as nonpublic hospitals become more particular about which charity cases they will admit. Such public hospitals have made modest efforts to reduce the amount of charitable care required of them, not so much by refusing patients as by urging voluntary hospitals to accept charity patients and to retain them rather than transfer them to the public hospital. Although isolated instances of success are reported, the trend data from 1980 show very little increase in charitable services by voluntary hospitals, so that large public hospitals have been forced to increase their provision of charitable care.[53] Presumably many of these hospitals will benefit from the Medicare adjustments under which hospitals with high indigent care burdens obtain extra payments.[54]

In large public teaching hospitals, the problems of uncompensated care are somewhat different. A substantial number of such hospitals, located in the nation's largest cities, have had very large charity and Medicare caseloads: 18 percent of charges in such hospitals have been due to charity and bad debt, in contrast to only 4.3 percent in voluntary teaching hospitals of comparable size.[55] Ironically, some of the nation's most expensive hospitals are teaching institutions that have been providing care to the nation's poorest people. For these hospitals the demise of cost shifting has become serious but thus far not life threatening. They have long covered uncompensated care through public subsidies and through their medical research and education funding. If they can retain sufficient public subsidies and education and research funds, they may be able to absorb most of the uncompensated care demands placed on them. To the extent that their research and education funds are imperiled or restricted, however, they will be less able to provide uncompensated care on their previous scale, and cuts in public spending that are not replaced by alternative programs will fall hard on their ability to serve the poor.[56]

Some parties have argued for identification and payment of the indirect and direct costs of medical education, so that society, especially the federal government, can better determine those costs and make more informed decisions about them. There is no reason, the argument runs, to bury the costs of medical education in reimbursement formulas for hospital care. It would be more prudent to sort out the costs of teaching. Consistently with this line of thought, some have argued that removing teaching costs from the Medicare program would help to delay insolvency in the Medicare trust fund. How much effect this would have on the future of Medicare is unclear, but such a change, in affecting the cost-shifting abilities of hospitals, would have a negative effect on care for the poor.[57]

Not all public teaching hospitals bear the same charity caseload. Ironically, the less the orientation of the public teaching hospital to the poor, the greater the stress resulting from diminished cost-shifting possibilities. In one sense, hospitals such as Cook County in Chicago are not adversely affected since for all practical purposes they never had patients who paid more than costs—although they are, of course, affected when the reduction of cost shifting causes other hospitals to dump patients on their doorstep. Large public hospitals that previously had numerous charge-paying patients, however, are seriously affected. The strategies open to such hospitals for coping with uncompensated care without cost shifting are essentially the same as those open to voluntary hospitals: persuade other hospitals to provide more charitable care, reduce charitable care, cut costs through greater efficiency, obtain more public funding for nonpaying patients, reincorporate in some fashion, or reduce programs.

The public nonteaching hospitals outside the largest cities, which are for many purposes not very different from voluntary hospitals, care for the poor in ways comparable to the voluntary sector. For the most part, their uncompensated care is small. Depending substantially on paying patients (whether Medicare or commercially insured), these hospitals will be squeezed moderately, if at all, as cost-shifting possibilities are curtailed. Unlike the three other kinds of public hospitals, these have more possibilities for entering into multi-institutional arrangements and for sharing services. As nonpublic hospitals reduce their uncompensated care, there may be pressure on these hospitals, as public institutions, to undertake more charity care.

Rural and small town public hospitals, already enormously pressed by low occupancy and with insufficient revenue to cover operating costs, are encountering additional financial stress because of the reduction in cost shifting. Although the percentage of patients who are paid for by Medicare is higher in urban than in rural areas, small public rural hospitals are quite dependent on Medicare for income. They have few Medicaid patients and budgets near zero for medical education and research, but they do carry charity caseloads that must be financed. Therefore, as changes in Medicare reimbursement have occurred and HMOs have reduced cost-shifting options, many small hospitals are facing yet another financial pressure to which they will find it difficult to respond.

Recognizing the difficulties of some small hospitals in isolated locations, the Health Care Financing Administration has made special exemptions for some of them in the DRG program. The exemptions, which apply to relatively few hospitals, are essentially directed to sole suppliers of hospital services in isolated areas.

Many small town and rural hospitals that do not qualify for special exemptions in the DRG program have complained strongly about the tremendous financial losses sustained as a result of the DRG Medicare reimbursement formula. Certainly many of them and their congressional representatives have made extremely vigorous efforts to slow the implementation of the DRG reimbursement program.[58]

The For-Profit Sector. As a general rule, the problems caused by curtailed cost shifting will be much less significant for proprietary hospitals, which have traditionally had small charity caseloads and very small roles in medical education and research. Thus most of the purposes for which cost shifting has been necessary in voluntary and public hospitals have been absent in for-profit hospitals. Most for-profit hospitals have served relatively few Medicaid patients and therefore have not shifted costs to cover Medicaid shortfalls. Moreover, most of them have had rather modest outpatient services. Outpatient services often lose money, especially if patients are paid for by Medicaid or by themselves. With their array of accountants and financial analysts, investor-owned hospital chains have been better able than other hospital organizations to adjust quickly to revenue changes and to modify their practices accordingly.

Usually not considered mainline community institutions, for-profit hospitals have greater flexibility to close departments and facilities that seem to require cost shifting. Although for-profit hospitals have generally admitted a higher percentage of emergency room clients than other hospitals, if they find that emergency facilities and emergency admissions are money losers, they can be expected to close them, secure in the knowledge that other hospitals provide such services. Some spokespersons for proprietary hospitals have suggested that their payment of taxes excuses them from any obligation to increase their uncompensated care—in contrast to voluntary hospitals, which enjoy a tax-exempt status.

Convergence: Projections

During most of the twentieth century, hospitals in the three sectors have become more alike, a trend largely to be explained by the greater similarity in their levels and sources of funding. Public hospitals, once swollen with almshouse caseloads and responsibilities, have spread throughout the United States, depending substantially on paying patients for revenue. Voluntary hospitals, once designed for the deserving poor, have moved from reliance on patients paying for their own care to reliance on patients paid for by public programs for over 50 percent of their budgets. For-profit hospitals, once wholly dependent on patients who paid directly for services, now derive about half their income from the same Medicare and Medicaid programs that support public and voluntary hospitals. These changes have led to greater similarity in behavior: more convergence in average bed size, more similarity in quality-oriented measures such as staffing and accreditation, more comparable facilities and services, and greater similarity in occupancy rates and length of stay.

The convergence of behavior among hospitals, especially between voluntary and for-profit hospitals, is not a subject about which there is universal agreement. One of the most articulate and insightful observers of the American hospital industry, Arnold Relman, has expressed considerable skepticism about the appropriateness of investor-owned hospitals. Yet he and other critics have often failed to acknowledge that voluntary hospitals, in much of their behavior, have become a mirror image of investor-owned hospitals. Of course, many scholars have pointed out that public hospitals, particularly in major cities, are still distinctive.

Observing considerable similarity in the recent behavior of hospitals of different kinds of ownership, some scholars have made the following policy recommendations, which are receiving considerable attention:

• that the tax advantages enjoyed by voluntary hospitals be reduced or eliminated on the grounds that they behave increasingly as for-profit hospitals do and that if any hospitals are to be tax exempt, it should be only because they provide specific services about which public authorities should be more explicit than they have been in recent decades

• that the return-on-equity advantages enjoyed by investor-owned hospitals in their Medicare reimbursement be reduced or eliminated on the grounds that voluntary hospitals, with the same business constraints, do not enjoy those benefits

• that the society cease to think of hospitals as voluntary, since almost all hospitals depend heavily on the public purse

• that we recognize that most hospitals seek to earn a profit, whose use and size vary from hospital to hospital (of course, the distribution of profits of hospitals legally designated as nonprofit has been constrained)

• that state governments implement all-payer systems so that hospitals receive sufficient funds to continue much of their education, research, and indigent care (an all-payer system recognizes that the financial needs of hospitals vary but should be based on the assumption that hospitals in certain classes have similar costs, irrespective of ownership)

• that even if an all-payer system is accepted, the society adopt some kind of insurance that will provide adequate care for those who face catastrophic medical costs and that if an all-payer system is rejected, the society explicitly provide funding for medical research and indigent care

Despite the recent trend toward convergence in American hospitals, the future of the hospital industry is one of considerable uncertainty. There is no certainty that the convergence will continue. Indeed, financial pressures on all kinds of hospitals will probably encourage them to become more differentiated rather than more alike. If the trend to convergence were reversed, society might well wish to preserve the special status of voluntary hospitals.

Able to distance themselves from public responsibilities and community pressures, investor-owned hospitals may increasingly become specialized centers for charge-paying patients. With profits somewhat less rewarding than in the very recent past, the growth of beds in investor-owned chains is slowing. Corporate owners may be quite happy to have their hospitals occupy relatively narrow niches as long as they bring adequate financial returns. If cost containment pressures become real enough, investor-owned hospitals may return to the marginal situation they occupied before the introduction of Medicare.

If this prospect of a retreat by proprietary hospitals is correct, public and voluntary hospitals would be left to provide most services for most patients. The extent of similarity of hospitals of comparable size would be conditioned by their levels and sources of funding. The behavior of voluntary and public hospitals, with half their revenue from Medicare and Medicaid and the other half mainly from commercially insured patients, would be much the same. But differences among hospitals in sources of revenue might begin to increase—some becoming more dependent on HMOs, the public purse, or well-financed third-party payers. And should variation in sources of revenue increase, differences in behavior would be expected to increase.

The few voluntary hospitals that might turn more sharply toward serving the poor would behave more like public hospitals in that their clients would be similar. Adequate reimbursement for caring for the poor should encourage similar behavior among recipient hospitals regardless of their ownership. The voluntary hospitals founded for religious reasons, located in large cities, and serving the poor are most likely to have a close resemblance to the public hospitals of major cities.

Many commentators fear that the nation is moving even more clearly to a two-tier system of hospitals, one tier providing high-quality, costly services to those with generous third-party benefits and the other providing low-quality, less expensive services to the underinsured and uninsured. This two-tier system might not be very different from the highly segmented, stratified system of the second and third decades of the twentieth century. If so, it would seem that American society has come full circle and that inequality in access to hospitals would remain very considerable.

The pressures to contain hospital costs may work to bring about a rationalization of care uncharacteristic of the American hospital sector. Hospitals, in their efforts to generate income to meet their expenses, may become true health centers, moving away from their exclusive dependency on acute-care specialization and assuming new roles in a continuum of care. So far, however, the cues for rationalization have

145

remained more theoretical than operative. The pressures to provide effective solutions for uncompensated care may be the key to instituting a form of planning hitherto notable by its absence. It seems more likely, however, that American hospitals will build on their history of patchwork institutions and funding, turning only modestly to the lessons of integration and linkage in other industries. Because of the intense competition and the lack of centralized control of the American medical system, it seems unlikely that it will become as coordinated as those in European countries, where the state has a much stronger role.

As long as American society chooses to finance medical care very much in the private sector and to treat various classes of patients differently, substantial differences in the behavior of hospitals will undoubtedly continue. Differences among hospitals of different kinds have narrowed when the society has made an effort to provide the same kind of treatment for all citizens, but society is not making a concerted effort to provide all Americans with equal access to medical care. At best, the result will probably be a halt in the trend to convergence in the hospital sector. Indeed, the behavior of hospitals with different kinds of ownership is likely to diverge if the number of Americans without any third-party coverage for medical care continues to increase.

Notes

1. Donald W. Light, "Corporate Medicine for Profit," *Scientific American*, vol. 255 (December 1986), p. 38.

2. Jo Ellen Mistarz, "The Changing Economic Profile of U.S. Hospitals," *Hospitals*, vol. 58 (May 16, 1984), pp. 83–88; Joyce Jensen and Ned Miklovic, "Declining Censuses Plague Hospitals; Administrators Expect Further Drops," *Modern Healthcare*, vol. 15 (August 16, 1985), pp. 86–87; and Karen Davis et al., "Is Cost Containment Working?" *Health Affairs*, vol. 4 (Fall 1985), pp. 81–94.

3. *Business Week*, January 12, 1987, p. 102.

4. Jack Hadley and Judith Feder, "Hospitals' Financial Status in 1980," Working Paper, Urban Institute, Washington, D.C., 1983, pp. 7–8.

5. *Wall Street Journal*, October 22, 1986.

6. Alan Sager, "Why Urban Voluntary Hospitals Close," *Health Services Research*, vol. 18 (Fall 1983), pp. 451–81; and "N.Y. City Has 25% Bed Surplus: State," *Modern Healthcare*, vol. 15 (August 26, 1985), p. 17.

7. *New York Times*, December 12, 1986; and Peter Salins, *New York Times*, January 31, 1987.

8. Davis et al., "Is Cost Containment Working?" pp. 89–90; *New York Times*, March 3, 1985; *Wall Street Journal*, March 18, 1985; and Sean Sullivan,

ed., *Managing Health Care Costs* (Washington, D.C.: American Enterprise Institute, 1984).

9. Jack Hadley and Judith Feder, "Hospitals' Financial Status and Care to the Poor in 1980: Executive Summary," Working Paper, Urban Institute, Washington, D.C., 1983, pp. 11–12.

10. Mistarz, "Changing Economic Profile," p. 88; Deborah Freko, "Admissions Fall but Margins Are Up in '84," *Hospitals*, vol. 59 (May 1, 1985), pp. 70–72.

11. *New York Times*, December 17, 1985; and *Business Week*, January 12, 1987, p. 102.

12. *Wall Street Journal*, December 4, 1986; and *New York Times*, March 29, 1987.

13. Ross Mullner, David L. McNeil, and Merwyn A. Landay, "Hospital Closures Remain Stable," *Hospitals*, vol. 59 (July 16, 1985), pp. 91–94; Ross Mullner, David L. McNeil, and Steven Andes, "National Trends in Hospital Closure, 1980–1984: A Description" (American Hospital Association, Office of Public Policy Analysis, Paper no. 54); Ross Mullner and David McNeil, "Closings Continue to Hit Smaller Hospitals," *Hospitals*, vol. 60 (April 5, 1986), p. 93; and A. Bruce Steinwald and Duncan Neuhauser, "The Role of the Proprietary Hospital," *Journal of Law and Contemporary Problems*, vol. 35 (1970), pp. 818–19.

14. Mark Tatge, "Occupancy Rate Declines Level Off While Outpatient Visits Continue Climb," *Modern Healthcare*, vol. 15 (May 10, 1985), p. 94; John Wennberg, Kim McPherson, and Philip Caper, "Will Payment Based on Diagnosis-related Groups Control Hospital Costs?" *New England Journal of Medicine*, vol. 311 (August 1984), pp. 295–300; Frank A. Sloan, Roger D. Feldman, and A. Bruce Steinwald, "Effects of Teaching on Hospital Costs," *Journal of Health Economics*, vol. 2 (1983), pp. 1–28; and Grace M. Carter and Paul B. Ginsburg, "The Medicare Case Mix–Index Increase: Medical Practice Changes, Aging, and DRG Creep," Report 3292-HCFA, Rand Corporation, June 1985.

15. Frank A. Sloan, "Property Rights in the Hospital Industry," in H. E. Frech III, ed., *Health Care in America: Political Economy of Hospitals and Health Insurance* (San Francisco: Pacific Research Institute for Public Policy, forthcoming).

16. Light, "Corporate Medicine," p. 42.

17. *Wall Street Journal*, January 22, 1987; and *New York Times*, April 16, 1986, and January 25, 1987.

18. Bill Jackson and Joyce Jensen, "Many Hospitals Report Census Drops; Workforces Haven't Felt Impact Yet," *Modern Healthcare*, vol. 14 (November 1, 1984), pp. 102–4.

19. Emily Friedman, "Indigent Care: Where the Marketplace Fails," *Hospitals*, vol. 59 (August 1, 1985), pp. 48–52; and Ruth Mintz, "Indigent Care Provider Fights for Fiscal Health," *Hospitals*, vol. 59 (August 1, 1985), pp. 53–54.

20. *Wall Street Journal*, November 11, 1980, and January 28, 1983.

21. William Shonick and Ruth Roemer, *Public Hospitals under Private Management* (Berkeley: Institute for Government Studies, University of California, 1983).

22. *New York Times,* July 23, 1986.

23. Salins, *New York Times,* January 31, 1987.

24. *New York Times,* November 3, 1986.

25. Marilyn Falik, "Hospital Financial Viability: When Is Government Intervention Appropriate?" *Health Services Research,* vol. 18 (Winter 1983), pp. 582–86.

26. "Public Hospital Buyouts Blocked," *Modern Healthcare,* vol. 13 (November 1983), p. 56.

27. *New York Times,* December 17, 1985.

28. *New York Times,* October 8, 10, 1985.

29. *Business Week,* January 12, 1987, p. 102.

30. Donald R. Cohodes, "Hospital Capital Formation in the 1980s: Is There a Crisis?" *Journal of Health Politics, Policy, and Law,* vol. 8 (Spring 1983), pp. 164–72.

31. M. A. Lightle and M. P. Plomann, "Hospital Capital Financing Entering Phase Four," *Hospitals,* vol. 55 (August 1, 1981), pp. 61–63; and Cohodes, "Hospital Capital Formation."

32. ICF, "An Analysis of Programs to Limit Hospital Capital Expenditures" (Washington, D.C.: Department of Health and Human Services, 1980), contract no. 233-79-3002, discussed in Cohodes, "Hospital Capital Formation."

33. J. Rogers Hollingsworth, *A Political Economy of Medicine: Great Britain and the United States* (Baltimore: Johns Hopkins University Press, 1986); Henry J. Aaron and William B. Schwartz, *The Painful Prescription: Rationing Hospital Care* (Washington, D.C.: Brookings Institution, 1984); and Brian Abel-Smith and Richard Titmuss, *The Cost of the National Health Service in England and Wales* (Cambridge: Cambridge University Press, 1956).

34. Unpublished statement by Robert H. Helms, acting assistant secretary of Department of Health and Human Services, presented to Subcommittee on Health, Committee on Finance, United States Senate, November 8, 1985. Hereafter cited as Helms, "Statement."

35. Patricia Arnold, "The Invisible Hand in Healthcare: The Rise of Markets within the U.S. Healthcare Sector" (Unpublished paper, University of Wisconsin, May 1986); United States General Accounting Office, "Hospital Merger Increased Medicare and Medicaid Payments for Capital Costs," Report to the Honorable Willis D. Gradison, Jr., House of Representatives (Washington, D.C., 1983).

36. Cohodes, "Hospital Capital Formation"; Arnold, "Invisible Hand"; and Helms, "Statement."

37. Interview with Leonard Marsh, Adventists Health System/Eastern and Middle America, March 1983. Marsh points out that Florida Southern Hospital in Orlando has taken the lead in obtaining bonding for seven small Adventist hospitals in Florida.

38. *New York Times,* January 13, 1987; and Robert O. Pasnau, "The Re-

medicalization of Psychiatry," *Hospital and Community Psychiatry,* vol. 38 (February 1987), p. 146.

39. Karen Davis and Diane Roland, "Uninsured and Underinsured: Inequities in Health Care in the United States," *Milbank Memorial Fund Quarterly,* vol. 61 (Spring 1983), pp. 149–76; Frank A. Sloan, Joseph Valvona, and Ross Mullner, "Identifying the Issues: A Statistical Profile," in Frank A. Sloan, James F. Blumstein, and James M. Perrin, eds., *Uncompensated Hospital Care: Defining Rights and Assigning Responsibilities* (Baltimore: Johns Hopkins University Press, 1983), p. 40.

40. *New York Times,* January 13, 1987, and March 14, 1987.

41. Ibid.; and *New York Times,* May 2, 1987.

42. The literature on cost shifting has become extensive. See Jack A. Meyer, *Passing the Health Care Buck* (Washington, D.C.: American Enterprise Institute, 1983); Charles E. Phelps, "Cross-Subsidies and Charge Shifting in American Hospitals," in Sloan, Blumstein, and Perrin, *Uncompensated Hospital Care;* Paul B. Ginsburg and Frank A. Sloan, "Hospital Cost Shifting," *New England Journal of Medicine,* vol. 310 (April 5, 1984), pp. 893–98; Sullivan, *Managing Health Care Costs;* and Barbara W. Greenman, *Cost Shifting: A Public Policy Debate* (Madison, Wis.: Institute for Health Planning, 1984).

43. Greenman, *Cost Shifting.*

44. Emily Friedman, "Shifting the Cost and the Blame," *Hospitals,* vol. 56 (March 16, 1983), pp. 93–97; Health Insurance Association of America, *Hospital Cost Shifting, the Hidden Tax: What Should Be Done about It* (Washington, D.C.: Hospital Insurance Association of America, 1982), pp. 4–5.

45. Hadley and Feder, "Hospitals' Financial Status."

46. Sloan, Valvona, and Mullner, "Identifying the Issues."

47. Robert M. Sigmond, "Selective Contracting and the Community Hospital," Michael M. Davis Lecture, Chicago, May 10, 1985; and Richard W. Foster, "The Nonprofit Hospital: Evolution and Future Prospects" (Unpublished paper, University of Colorado at Denver, September 1983).

48. Rosemary A. Stevens, "Voluntary and Governmental Activity," *Health Matrix,* vol. 3 (Spring 1985), pp. 26–31; and Sigmond, "Selective Contracting."

49. A. Relman, "The New Medical-Industrial Complex," *New England Journal of Medicine,* vol. 303 (1980), pp. 963–68; Rosemary Stevens, "The Changing Hospital," in Linda H. Aiken and David Mechanic, eds., *Applications of Social Science to Clinical Medicine Health Policy* (New Brunswick, N.J.: Rutgers University Press, 1986), pp. 80–99; and H. Hansmann, "The Role of Nonprofit Enterprise," *Yale Law Journal,* vol. 89 (1980), pp. 835–43.

50. *New York Times,* May 25, 1986.

51. Jack A. Meyer, "Financing Uncompensated Care with All-Payer Rate Regulation," in Sloan, Blumstein, and Perrin, *Uncompensated Hospital Care.*

52. *Wall Street Journal,* March 31, 1987.

53. Judith Feder, Jack Hadley, and Ross Mullner, "Falling through the Cracks: Poverty, Insurance Coverage, and Hospital Care for the Poor, 1980 and 1982," *Health and Society,* vol. 62 (1984), pp. 544–66.

54. *Wall Street Journal,* March 31, 1987.

55. Sloan, Valvona, and Muller, "Identifying the Issues," p. 23.

56. Testimony of Dr. James D. Bentley of the Association of Medical Colleges before U.S. House of Representatives, Ways and Means Committee, Subcommittee on Health, *Issues Relating to Medicare Hospital Payments*, May 14, 1985.

57. See U.S. House of Representatives, Committee on Ways and Means, *Deficit Reduction Amendments of 1985: Report to Accompany H.R. 3128, Dissenting and Additional Dissenting Views*, Report 99-141, pt. I, July 31, 1985.

58. Testimony before U.S. House of Representatives, Ways and Means Committee, Subcommittee on Health, *Issues Relating to Medicare Hospital Payments*, May 14, 1985.

Appendix:
Concepts and Data

Concepts

Size. Size is a variable often overlooked in social science research, but we believe that it greatly influences the behavior of organizations, and considerable literature suggests that the size of hospitals varies with the type of ownership.[1] For this reason we discuss how size, other behavioral characteristics, type of ownership, and source of funding are interrelated.

Costs and Profits. We would prefer to measure the efficiency of hospitals, but social scientists have not been very successful in measuring hospital efficiency.[2] As a result we confine our attention to measuring the operating costs of hospitals per bed, per patient day, and per admission. We also report the margin, or profit (that is, the difference between expenses and revenues).

Equality of Access by Social Classes and Income Groups. Although equality is defined in many different ways in the scholarly literature, our concern is simply to determine whether public sector and private sector hospitals provide services to essentially the same or to different social classes or groups.[3] By analyzing data longitudinally, it is possible to determine whether public sector, voluntary, and for-profit institutions tend over time to provide essentially the same services to all social classes or groups. Fortunately, we have a number of studies on which to build.[4]

Utilization. Utilization refers in this study to the extent to which hospitals keep their beds full and how rates of occupancy are related to different case mixes. The extent to which higher occupancy is associated with longer average stay is an important dimension of utilization. Utilization also refers to the extent to which hospitals in different sectors are providing outpatient (including emergency) services.

151

Quality of Medical Services. By definition, quality is concerned with the effect of care on the health of the individual. Attempts to measure health care quality are usually of three kinds: evaluation of structure, evaluation of process, and evaluation of outcomes. Such things as physical aspects of facilities and equipment are structural indicators, as are characteristics of the organization and qualifications of health professionals. Measures of process are such things as the activities of health professionals in patient care. Outcome may be measured by health or by satisfaction.[5]

Numerous researchers have attempted to develop a reliable index of the quality of hospital care in terms of final outcomes, but thus far scholars have viewed outcome measures with considerable skepticism in evaluating hospital performance.[6] Partly for this reason, much of the scholarly literature simply ignores the issue of quality. It appears, however, that case-related data connected with the use of diagnosis-related groups (DRGs) for Medicare may provide much fuller data of higher quality than have previously been available. A few outcome analyses are now available.[7]

To confront these problems Newhouse and Feldstein have provided a logical argument for the use of inputs as a proxy for quality.[8] No single input characteristic, however, is an adequate measure of all inputs or of the quality of hospital medical services, and for this reason our strategy is to use several measures. In doing so, we measure different dimensions of quality, for quality of medical services is a multidimensional concept. The dimensions we propose to use are quality of staff and quality of standards employed in the hospital.

We measure quality of staff by the number of full-time-equivalent employees per bed, a measure frequently used in the literature.[9] For some years we also report the number of interns and residents for each hospital. The quality of standards employed in the hospital is measured by whether it has received accreditation from the Joint Commission on the Accreditation of Hospitals or the American College of Surgeons.

Technological Complexity. Technological complexity refers to the extent to which hospitals in different sectors offer more complex and differentiated services, usually made possible through the addition of sophisticated equipment and facilities and of highly trained professional staff. The more facilities and services a hospital offers, the greater the extent to which it can provide intensive and specialized care, rather than basic care with ancillary services.

152

Data

The 1935 data are from the Business Census of Hospitals, carried out by the U.S. Public Health Service in 1935 with the aid of grants from the Works Progress Administration. The major publications resulting from this census were these:

1. *Business Census of Hospitals, 1935: General Report*, by Elliott H. Pennell, Joseph Mountin, and Kay Pearson. Published as Supplement No. 154 to the *Public Health Reports*.
2. *Hospital Facilities in the United States*
"Selected Characteristics of Hospital Facilities in 1936," by Joseph W. Mountin, Elliott H. Pennell, and Evelyn Flack.
"Trends in Hospital Development, 1928–1936," by Joseph W. Mountin, Elliott H. Pennell, and Kay Pearson.
Public Health Bulletin, no. 243 (September 1938).
3. "Prevailing Ratios of Personnel to Patients in Hospitals Offering General Care," by Elliott H. Pennell, Joseph W. Mountin, and Kay Pearson, *Hospitals*, vol. 12 (November 1938), pp. 42–47.
4. "Summary Figures on Income, Expenditures, and Personnel of Hospitals," by Elliott H. Pennell, Joseph W. Mountin, and Emily Hankla, *Hospitals*, vol. 12 (April 1938), pp. 11–17. This article was adapted and published as "Summary Figures on Income, Expenditures, and Personnel of Hospitals," same authors, in *The Hospital in Modern Society*, edited by Arthur C. Bachmeyer and Gerhard Hartman (New York: Commonwealth Fund, 1943), pp. 65–78.
5. "The Financial Support of Non-Government Hospitals as Revealed by the Recent Federal Business Census of Hospitals," by Elliott H. Pennell and Joseph W. Mountin, *Hospitals*, vol. 11 (December 1937), pp. 11–19.

Although all these publications have the same data base, they report slightly different findings, evidently because of decisions about dropping observations with missing data and estimating missing data. We have adopted the convention, in instances in which different data are reported, of using the value based on the largest number of observations.

The 1939 report *Hospital and Other Institutional Facilities and Services, 1939 (Vital Statistics*, Special Reports, Bureau of the Census, vol. 13, September 15, 1941) found that although about 18.4 percent of hospitals were not registered and were thus omitted from the 1935–1936 survey, the omitted hospitals accounted for a very small portion of patient activities (1.7 percent of days of care).

The 1961 data are drawn from the American Hospital Association (AHA) annual survey. These data were made available in published form and as a machine-readable data tape.

The following procedures were observed in using the data tape:

• Analysis was confined to short-term general hospitals in the United States for which the number of statistical beds had been determined by the AHA.

• Variables from the data tape that were used without modification are adult beds, bassinets, accreditation by the Joint Commission on the Accreditation of Hospitals, and interns and residents.

• A score for each hospital was derived by summing the number of facilities and services in the AHA survey, omitting chest X-ray on admission, organized hospital auxiliary, and chapel or prayer room. The maximum number of facilities and services was twenty-one.

There were 5,042 hospitals used in this analysis.

The 1979 data are also drawn from the AHA annual survey, both the published form and the machine-readable data tape. The number of hospitals used in the analysis was 5,750. The procedures for 1979 followed those used for 1961 except that the maximum score on the facilities and services scale was forty-three. Items omitted from the scale (but included in the survey) were volunteer services departments, patient representative services, and hospital auxiliaries.

Notes

1. Rosemary Stevens, *American Medicine and the Public Interest* (New Haven, Conn.: Yale University Press, 1971); and Bruce Steinwald and Duncan Neuhauser, "The Role of the Proprietary Hospital," *Journal of Law and Contemporary Problems*, vol. 35 (1970), pp. 817–35.

2. Allan S. Detsky, *The Economic Foundations of National Health Policy* (Cambridge, Mass.: Ballinger, 1978). See also Frank Sloan, "Property Rights in the Hospital Industry," in H. E. Frech III, ed., *Health Care in America: Political Economy of Hospitals and Health Insurance* (San Francisco: Pacific Research Institute for Public Policy, forthcoming). The Sloan study is a review of much of the recent literature on efficiency and costs.

3. J. Rogers Hollingsworth, "Inequality in Levels of Health in England, 1891–1971," *Journal of Health and Social Behavior*, vol. 22 (September 1981), pp. 268–83.

4. Karen Davis, "Economic Theories of Behavior in Non-Profit, Private Hospitals," *Economics and Business Bulletin*, vol. 24 (Winter 1972), pp. 1–13; Milton I. Roemer and Jorge Mera, "Patient Dumping and Other Voluntary Agency Contributions to Public Agency Problems," *Medical Care*, vol. 11 (January–February 1973), pp. 30–39; and J. Rogers Hollingsworth, *A Political*

Economy of Medicine: Great Britain and the United States (Baltimore: Johns Hopkins University Press, 1986).

5. David D. Rutstein et al., "Measuring the Quality of Medical Care," *New England Journal of Medicine*, vol. 294 (March 11, 1976), pp. 582–88; see also discussion in Committee on Implications of For-Profit Enterprise in Health Care, Institute of Medicine, Bradford H. Gray, ed., *For-Profit Enterprise in Health Care* (Washington, D.C.: National Academy Press, 1986), chap. 6, pp. 127–41.

6. Gary Gaumer, "Medicare Patient Outcomes and Hospital Organizational Mission," in Gray, *For-Profit Enterprise*, pp. 354–74. See also Victor R. Fuchs, *The Health Economy* (Cambridge, Mass.: Harvard University Press, 1986).

7. Milton I. Roemer, A. Taher Moustafa, and Cara F. Hopkins, "A Proposed Hospital Quality Index: Hospital Death Rates Adjusted for Case Severity," *Health Services Research*, vol. 3 (Summer 1968), pp. 113–17.

8. Joseph Newhouse, "Toward a Theory of Nonprofit Institutions: An Economic Model of a Hospital," *American Economic Review*, vol. 60 (1970), pp. 64–73; and Martin S. Feldstein, "Hospital Cost Inflation: A Study of Non-Profit Price Dynamics," *American Economic Review*, vol. 61 (1971), pp. 853–72.

9. Detsky, *Economic Foundations*.

Index

ACS. *See* American College of Surgeons
Acute-care hospitals. *See* Community
   hospitals
All-payer system, 40, 53, 144
Almshouses, 42–43
AMA. *See* American Medical Association
American College of Surgeons, 45–46,
   61, 95
American Hospital Association, 31, 35
American Medical Association, 61, 95
American Medical International, 66–67
AMI. *See* American Medical International
Arrow, Kenneth, 4, 63

Behavior, hospital. *See* Hospital behavior
Blue Cross
   features, 31
   history, 31–33
   role, 32
Boston City Hospital, 43, 44, 46–47
Brooklyn Hospital, 28

Capital
   improvements, 12, 92
   needs, 41, 132–33, 135, 136
   sources, 9, 28–29, 30, 33–34, 41–42,
     89–91, 92
Care, uncompensated, 40, 92, 93, 106,
   107, 116, 136–43
Certificate of need. *See* Regulation,
   certificate of need
Charity Hospital (New Orleans), 45
Community hospitals, 18–19, 34, 51, 70,
   99, 102. *See also* Investor-owned
   hospitals; Public hospitals; Voluntary
   hospitals
CON. *See* Regulation, certificate of need
Consolidation, 9–10, 12–13, 40, 73, 134
Convergence, 13–15, 143–46
Cook County Hospital (Chicago), 43, 46–
   47, 48, 141
Costs. *See also* Investor-owned hospitals;
   Public hospitals; Voluntary hospitals
   Blue Cross and, 32
   Medicare and, 35–37, 38

regulations and, 38–40, 144
   sunk, 27
Cost shifting, 40, 137–38, 140, 141, 142–
   43
Cross-subsidization. *See* Cost shifting

Demand, nature of, 49–50
Depression, 49, 61
Diagnosis-related groups, 39–40, 67, 70,
   126–27, 135
   uncompensated care and, 140, 142
DRGs. *See* Diagnosis-related groups

Economies of scale, 9–10, 40, 65
Education, medical, 47–48, 65, 109, 141

Facilities and services. *See* Technological
   complexity
Federal government. *See also* Regulation
   diagnosis-related groups and, 39–40
   Hill-Burton Act and, 33–34, 49
   medical policies, 37–38

Groups, diagnosis-related. *See* Diagnosis-
   related groups

HCA. *See* Hospital Corporation of
   America
Health maintenance organizations
   (HMOs), 126, 128, 131–32, 138
Hill-Burton Act, 35, 96–99, 103
   effects, 50, 51
   history, 7–8, 33–34, 49–50
   purpose, 33
HMOs. *See* Health maintenance
   organizations
Homer G. Phillips Hospital (St. Louis),
   53
Hospital behavior
   changes over time, 41–42, 116–17
   comparison (of sectors), 13–15, 45,
     63, 86–87, 116–19, 143
   indicators of, 88–89
   in 1935, 89–96
   in 1961, 96–102

157

160

A NOTE ON THE BOOK

This book was edited by Trudy Kaplan of the
Publications Staff of the American Enterprise Institute.
The index was prepared by Julia Stam.
The text was set in Palatino, a typeface designed by Hermann Zapf.
Coghill Book Typesetting Company, of Richmond, Virginia,
set the type, and Edwards Brothers Incorporated,
of Ann Arbor, Michigan, printed and bound the book,
using permanent, acid-free paper.

WITHDRAWN

DATE DUE

GAYLORD			PRINTED IN U.S.A.